BACK together

Hands-On Healing for Couples

by Andrew S. Kirschner, D.O.

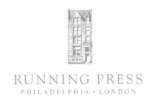

RUNNING PRESS
PHILADELPHIA · LONDON

© 2005 by Andrew S. Kirschner, D.O.
© 2005 Photography by Gregory Katz

All rights reserved under the Pan-American and International Copyright Conventions
Printed in China

9 8 7 6 5 4 3 2 1

Digit on the right indicates the number of this printing

Library of Congress Control Number 2005902523

ISBN 13: 978-0-7624-2403-0
ISBN 10: 0-7624-2403-6

Cover and interior designed by Corinda Cook
Edited by Sheridan McCarthy
Photography by Gregory Katz and Andrew S. Kirschner, except photographs on pages 62 and 82 © Photodisc by Getty Images.
Typography: Caslon and Trade Gothic

This book may be ordered by mail from the publisher. Please include $2.50 for postage and handling.
But try your bookstore first!

Running Press Book Publishers
125 South Twenty-second Street
Philadelphia, Pennsylvania 19103-4399

Visit us on the web!
www.runningpress.com

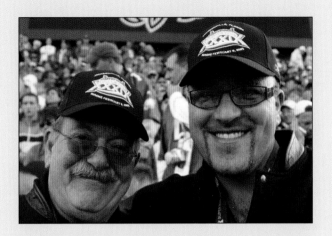

To the best Physician I know, my dad.
Your knowledge, wisdom, and love have
given me the tools to achieve my dreams.

Contents

Part One: The Talk

Part Two: The Walk

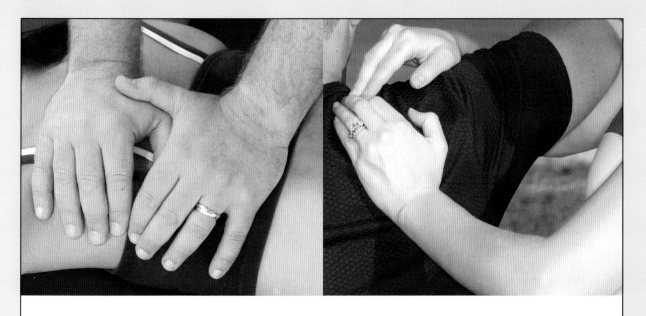

Part Three: The Lifestyle

Foreword

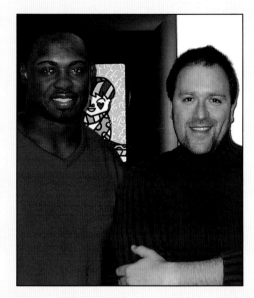

When I first hurt my back in 1999, I thought it would be like a lot of the injuries that I've had playing this game called football. I thought it would hurt for a while and then one day just stop, as if by magic. But of course, it didn't. The pain didn't go away, and it began to affect my daily life. The first thing I noticed was how hard it was getting up and down from the floor to play with my children. I also noticed the pain I felt doing simple things like picking up five or six bags of groceries or a full load of laundry at once and lugging them up the steps. I could do these things, but it always cost me later.

Other fatherly pleasures such as piggyback rides for my kids, push-ups with them on my back, and long rides on daddy's shoulders were cut to a minimum. I could take pain medication, but I realized the drugs only hid the problem. (The best analogy I've heard is that pain medication is like a fire chief sending an entire fire department to a roaring fire only to have them spray water on the fire alarms.)

Of course, back pain had an effect on my job. Not only did the pain in my back restrict some of my movements, it caused other things to go wrong. Simple things, such as just getting in a football stance, back peddling, sudden change in directions, and one of my favorites—making big hits— were all compromised. I still could do them, but not to the best of my ability.

Because my job required me to do all of the above, I felt compelled to fight through the pain and, of course, I suffered the consequences, which was that other parts of my back began to join in the fun, causing me more pain to fight through. There were times when my entire back would feel like an award-winning choir with all the members singing all the time. In addition, I was forcing other parts of my body to overcompensate, such as my hamstrings, my groin area, my traps, and my calves. I would find out later that a lot of the pulls and strains I had in my muscles during that time were directly the result of my back pain left untreated.

The greatest cost was at home with my family, where—unlike at work—I didn't have to force myself to fight through the pain. Some days I could barely move. I was playing with my kids and helping around the house less and less. Worst of all, having quality time with my wife was very near impossible because I felt miserable so much of the time. Eventually I realized that I was making my wife and kids miserable as well, and I knew I could not go on like this. The most important thing in my life is my family, but I had allowed back pain to make me put them last.

A very fortunate thing happened then. A friend referred me to Dr. Kirschner, or "The Fix," as I like to call him. Up until then, I'd avoided "back doctors" because the treatments I'd heard about worried me. Painful hard crunches and surgery that took months to recover from were not what I wanted.

Right away, I knew Dr. K was different from other doctors I'd seen. He told me that many of football players, who regularly get beaten up a lot, couldn't take hard crunches, so he created a gentler treatment plan that was painless and effective, and didn't involve lots of prescriptions. For the first time, I had someone telling me that it was possible to live without pain, without being hooked on pills, or going under the knife.

He also asked me questions about how my back was affecting my home life —not just my work—and was not surprised to hear that my family, particularly my wife, was suffering because of my chronic pain. Dr. K explained that many of his patients had similar stories, and that often the stress at home made people's pain feel even worse, causing a vicious cycle of pain, stress, and more pain. He encouraged me to bring my wife in so she could better understand my pain and my treatment, including her in the process and working on her own back pain as well. Dr. K's techniques have been really helpful to both of us, and understanding the treatment has helped us connect better.

When I leave Dr. K's office on Saturday before the Sunday game, I know my body is in full readiness to play, and that I'm likely to come home without feeling wrecked because I've pushed myself too far. My mind and body feel prepared to go out and be the best, both on the field and at home. Working with Dr. K has helped me to be a better player on my team, a better father to my kids, and, most importantly, a better husband to my wife.

The life of a professional football player is necessarily about dealing with pain. I feel blessed to have found a solution for some of it. After reading this book and learning Dr. K's techniques, I know you will feel blessed as well.

Brian Dawkins

Philadelphia Eagles

Acknowledgments

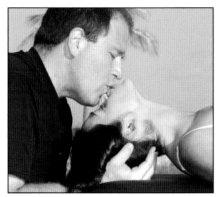

Thank you. Thank you. Thank you:

Mom, you are amazing! Thank you for believing.

Donna, *Back Together* wouldn't exist without you. Thanks for propping me up when I feel like falling down, and kicking me in the butt when I slack off. You have taught me so much about so many things. I love you.

To my daughter Ella, carrying you lightens my load.

Julie, your keen eye and open ears have helped see this project through.

Clifford, Peter, Eric, and the rest of my family, you've been there for me in more ways than you will ever know.

Rose and Kevin, you have helped to make a really cool mountain out of a solid molehill.

To Drs. Young, Big Nick, and all of the teachers who inspired me to pursue my dream—thanks.

Clarence and Jorden—see you in Miami!

Lauree and Greg, thanks for making me look good.

Danielle, thanks for putting out the fires. You're a great assistant and wonderful friend.

Deborah, you made me feel like a real author.

Brian and Connie—what can I say? You are both wonderful.

To all of my friends, patients and readers: Your love, support, and trust mean the world to me.

Most sincerely,

Andy

P.S.: Thanks to those folks at that ubiquitous coffee store who kept me pumped up with countless Venti black iced teas and tolerated my **omnipresence**. Your caffeine keeps me good and jittery.

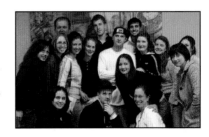

This is Not a Self-Help Book . . .

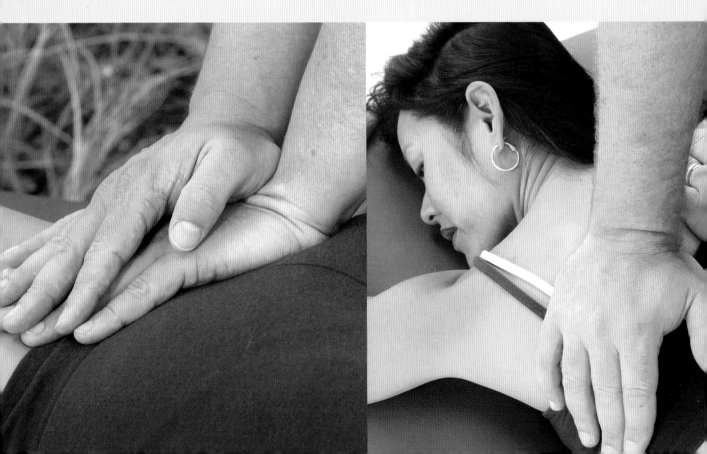

I hate self-help books.

There, I said it. I told a friend I was going to write a book about musculoskeletal pain, and how to deal with it or even get rid of it, and he said sarcastically, "Oh boy! Another self-help book! Yeah, that's exactly what you need to do. I'll go get the incense and crystals." I didn't understand what he meant by the comment, because up until this point I had not really read any "self-help" books.

I went to my local bookstore, sat down on the floor, and read for about five hours. From depression to financial freedom, and even to back pain: I read, took notes, and determined that I would not write a self-help book.

All of the books I read that day suggested that the authors had special knowledge or a magical ingredient that allowed them to provide the reader with a spectacular cure-all for whatever they were writing about. I have no doubt that their information was helpful and productive more often than not, but I want to make it clear from the start that I do not possess any secret potions, charms, spells, magical powers, or divine inspiration. I am not a guru. I don't suggest that through some sleight of hand I will miraculously make your pain go away. I am simply a physician who has had the good fortune to treat many patients for their pain. I have spent a great deal of time and energy observing what works and what doesn't. I have worked with every type of body, from professional athletes at the peak of conditioning to the physically disabled, from newborn infants to the elderly. I have looked at everyone's approaches, gadgets, and manuals, selected what I think offers the most benefit, and added my own ideas. The

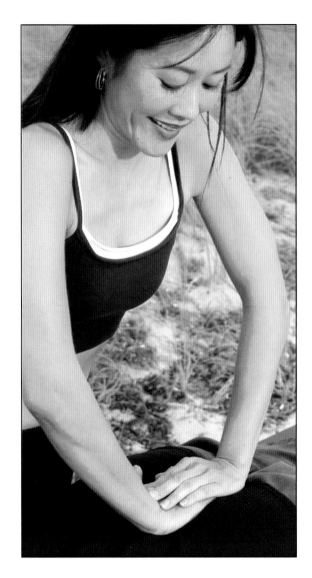

techniques I outline for you will not work on everyone, but will probably help most.

I created this program to use as a toolbox for *couples*, because we often forget that the pain sufferer's partner often suffers almost as much, albeit in different ways. We physicians tend to think of our patients as alone (the way we often see them in our offices), and only in terms of their current complaints. In my practice I have seen the devastating effects of pain on relationships; the spouse or partner often develops feelings of frustration, anger, and helplessness in the face of their loved one's plight. I have seen that a partner's skilled application of these techniques can offer greater and longer-lasting benefit than when they are applied by a physician or therapist. I want to offer both partners several approaches that will empower them to take an active role in their well-being, and offer them the opportunity I enjoy every day—to help each other to feel better. As I said earlier, your partner is often your best resource for beginning to heal— after all, who else has a bigger stake in your feeling better?

At one time or another, most people experience some sort of musculoskeletal pain, and these tools can help them and their partners minimize the damage. I don't expect you to experience any sort of revelation or epiphany. I simply wish to help you and your partner understand the mechanics of pain: what causes it, what helps treat it, what helps prevent it. Then we will develop strategies for eliminating its effects from your daily lives as much as possible. The rewards can be astounding!

You can take a look at the contents of this toolbox, and use those techniques that you think will apply to the situation that the two of you are in.

To make the underlying concepts accessible, I describe them using a minimum of technical or medical terminology. If you have a medical background, some descriptions may sound simplistic; however, I urge you to give them a read anyway because they may actually help you think about these conditions in ways you haven't before.

Introducing A Partner-Based Approach

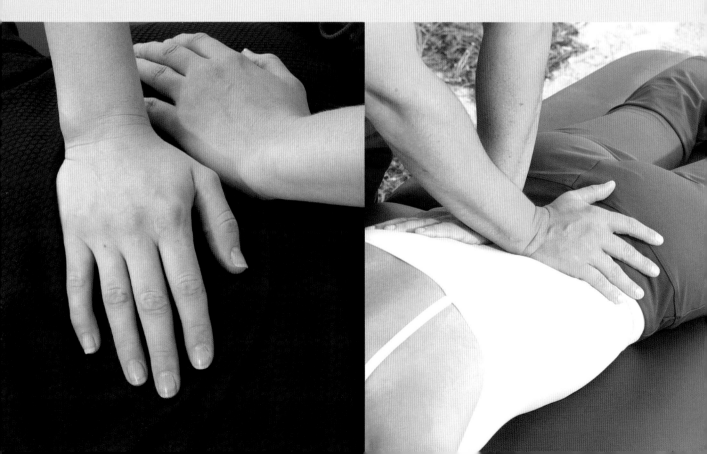

I was inspired to create the partner-based approach to back pain during one of the most amazing moments of my life—the birth of my daughter. My wife Donna and I had both decided that it would be beneficial for our daughter to come into the world peacefully and without medication. During labor, I applied some basic soft tissue maneuvers to her spine, and relieved a significant amount of her labor discomfort. If you have delivered children of your own, you can appreciate that this is no small feat. She had a relatively comfortable birth. The nursing staff in her delivery room kept asking what I had done to help Donna—was I sneaking her pills? Had I used some voodoo spell to help her through her pain?

Donna, herself a childbirth educator, asked me how complicated it would be to integrate some of the techniques I had applied during her labor into her own childbirth classes—to offer partners of the mothers-to-be the opportunity to have a direct, hands-on impact on the labor experience. We quickly found that this not only helped the mother to have a more comfortable labor, but also allowed the partner to feel like a more integrated contributor to the birthing experience.

I expanded the techniques to include maneuvers and strategies that could be applied by virtually anyone to help deal with back and neck pain. I taught them to couples among my patients, and they were thrilled with the results they could achieve on their own. With some practice, they experienced better, longer-lasting results than with my treatments alone. I attribute this difference to the energy and chemistry that loved ones share, which could never be replicated in a clinical setting.

I created *Back Together* in response to what I perceived as three big problems people face when dealing with back and neck pain. First and foremost, there is an education gap. Literally millions of people walking around in pain every day know the *name* of their diagnosis, but do not understand what that name really means. I believe that if people understand the mechanism of their pain, they will be much better equipped to reduce their risk of injury and help themselves feel better. Second, back pain affects virtually every aspect of the sufferer's life, and can have a profound emotional effect on his sense of well-being. In my experience, a person empowered with tools to help control his own pain has a better quality of life than one who continuously depends upon physicians and therapists. Last, I found that the entire medical model ignores a fundamental element in the chain of recovery—the partners of those in pain. We all understand the ways in which the life of the pain sufferer is affected, but his partner often suffers as well, in complex and destructive ways. **By bringing a partner into the recovery picture, we can facilitate healing for both partners, and offer them something truly special—the ability to help heal one another.**

What You'll Learn

Since musculoskeletal pain comes from many sources, I have produced a multifaceted approach to address its causes, and then help relieve it. The hands-on techniques you will learn are largely based on the principles of Osteopathic Medicine. (You may notice the prefix "osteo" popping up a lot in this book. "Osteo" simply refers to bony structures.) They are also drawn from such disciplines as myofascial release, shiatsu, acupressure, and cranial-sacral work. For this book, the techniques will primarily deal with pain in what we refer to as the axial skeleton—your head, neck, and mid- and low back. I will touch upon the basics of Osteopathy shortly.

Bear in mind, hands-on techniques are only a small piece of the picture. By addressing some of the psychological and lifestyle issues I discuss, you will greatly increase the likelihood of improvement.

It is extremely important that you understand that **the techniques in this book are not designed to treat or cure any condition**. They are designed to improve the function of individuals in discomfort, and to hopefully reduce the effect of pain on their daily lives.

I have divided the rest of this book into several sections:

The Talk

- The basic anatomy and physiology of pain.

- The triad of pain, and how its elements feed each other to reinforce the cycle of pain.

- The psychological effects of pain.

- Retraining your body to function without pain.

The Walk

- Guidelines to follow when trying the techniques.

- Learning the basics of Orthokinetic Soft Tissue Optimization.

- 16 effective hands-on techniques to try.

The Lifestyle

- How ergonomics play a part in pain and recovery.

- The importance of exercise and other lifestyle habits.

- The fit of your clothes—an overlooked factor in pain.

I will encourage you to ask yourself questions. Your answers will often be surprising and dictate the direction you will take. Please note that I wrote this as though I were speaking to both you and your partner, so I alternate gender throughout the book.

I hope you enjoy the *incredibly fabulous* anecdotes I have included in an effort to keep this dry topic from becoming desert-like. I wish to thank you from the bottom of my heart for wanting to listen to what I have to say.

My Love Affair with Osteopathic Medicine

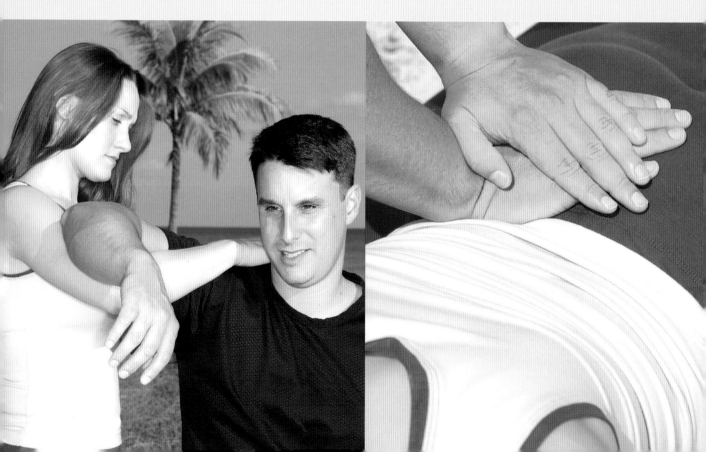

When I was 14, my grandfather went to his family doctor for back pain. The doctor told him that it was arthritis, a normal consequence of his age, and that anti-inflammatory medication would be his best course of treatment. When the pain became worse, he was prescribed pain medication and muscle relaxants. When these ceased to be effective, the doctor ordered narcotics.

The x-rays were unremarkable, and the doctor was at a loss to explain why Grandpa's back hurt so badly. My father, also a physician, asked my grandfather if he would be willing to see a doctor we all knew as "Big Nick." Everyone regarded Dr. Nicholas as a miracle worker, one of a dying breed of old-school Osteopaths—the one everyone went to as a last resort. If anyone could solve the mystery of my grandfather's pain, it would be him.

When Big Nick came into the room, it quickly became apparent why he possessed such a colorful nickname; Nicholas Nicholas, D.O. was an enormous man with an enormous personality. He sat down and they began to review Grandfather's symptoms: back pain localized to one area below his right shoulder blade. No injury or trauma preceded this pain, and the supposed "arthritis" had mysteriously missed every other joint in his body.

Big Nick placed his gigantic hands on my grandfather's back, and scanned across, up, and down, as though he were reading a newspaper in Braille. This continued for about a minute; then he said to my grandfather, "There's something going on in the head of your pancreas. I cannot say that I know exactly what it is, but that's *where* it is." He recommended a CT scan of his abdomen.

When the results of the scan came back a few days later, we learned that there was evidence of a 1-centimeter tumor in the head of the pancreas. Pancreatic cancer is about the most aggressive cancer there is, more often than not a certain death sentence. Even today, most patients survive approximately six months following the discovery of the cancer.

Even though I had grown up in a medical family, my exposure to death and dying was basically nonexistent at fourteen. My grandfather and I were very close and his death several months later profoundly affected me, guiding many of my career choices thereafter.

When I started applying to medical schools, my father, an Osteopathic ear, nose, and throat surgeon, strongly encouraged me to pursue an M.D. degree instead of the D.O. degree I was ultimately to receive. D.O.s were still subject to prejudice outside the Philadelphia region where we lived, and he thought I would have an easier time in an M.D.'s world than in his. When I asked Big Nick, he recalled the day in his office when he used his hands to diagnose something that my grandfather's own internist dismissed as a normal consequence of aging. I had always wondered if an earlier diagnosis could have changed the out-

come. I know now that it probably would not, but beginning that day, I focused on getting into a good Osteopathic school.

Since graduating in 1995, I have had the good fortune to work with some of the most talented Osteopathic physicians in the world. When I finally made it through medical school, internship, residency, and a brief stay in a medical practice that confirmed for me everything I thought was wrong with medicine, I opened my own practice. I was told that going into private practice was crazy—but lo and behold, people came and my practice grew. I started getting referrals from referrals, and I knew that the things I did worked. People came to me in pain and left feeling better. It could take days, weeks, or occasionally longer, but patients really responded to the treatment style I was slowly developing.

Brian Dawkins, one of the best players in the NFL, was referred to my practice and became a regular client. Soon, my office became a "pregame clinic" on Saturdays, and Eagles' players getting a tune-up often encountered players who had come to town to play against them the next day. Word spread to other professional athletes, and before I knew it, players from around the NFL and other sports were coming to me for relief from their pain. I received requests to go to Europe, and even had the opportunity to treat royalty.

As word spread and my practice grew, I was smiling inside, not only because I was helping so many people, but also because I knew that the techniques I was using were so simple. The true magic was that *there was no magic*! I knew that anyone could learn methods for preventing, reducing, and often eliminating pain. I don't say that these methods are a panacea, but I do believe that when properly applied, they can vastly improve an individual's quality of life.

I have applied these hands-on procedures to my patients, my friends, and my family. I know they work—and work well. When I implement these techniques, I can facilitate healing. I can reduce pain. I can restore function. And when a person uses the same techniques properly on a loved one, they tend to work even better.

I hope that by learning and practicing some of the maneuvers outlined in this book, along with the strategies and suggestions I will present, you will derive some of the satisfaction I have had when I use my hands to help people feel better.

When Your Wife's Masseuse Looks Like Ricky Martin

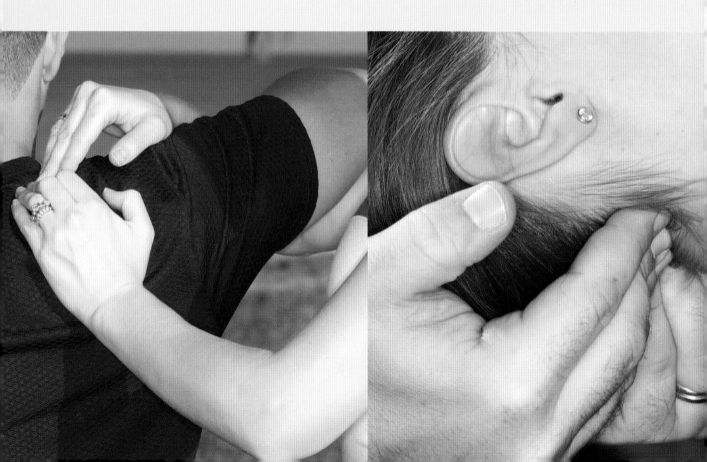

As I related earlier, I created *Back Together* to empower couples by giving them the tools they need to help think about pain, to help reduce it, and to help prevent it in the first place. In practice, however, many individuals still depend on professionals to help with some aspects of their pain management. Here is an example of one of the ways this dependency upon professionals can go terribly wrong.

Rachel and Kurt (not their real names, which are Debby and Larry) had been dealing with Rachel's low back pain for some time. Rachel found that a massage every few weeks went a long way towards helping her remain functional and in a pain-reduced state.

Over several months, Rachel received regular massage therapy from a very talented therapist named Steve. Kurt decided to get a massage himself and scheduled with Steve. My conversation with Kurt the day after his appointment went something like this:

Kurt: "Hey Andy, I got my massage from Steve last night."

Me: "Yeah, how'd it go?"

Kurt: "Pretty good, I think—did you know Steve looks an awful lot like Ricky Martin?"

Me: "Yes, I guess he sort of does."

Kurt: "I know it shouldn't bother me, but I'm not all that thrilled that my wife is getting felt up by this guy every week."

Me: "Well, you know he *is* a professional; I don't think it's the same thing as being 'felt up.' I wouldn't let it bother you too much—Rachel is in love with you."

Kurt: "I know, I know, but I wonder if she would feel as good if he didn't look like Ricky Martin."

Me: "I honestly don't think that has much to do with it. He's a good massage therapist. I've sent plenty of male and female patients to him and he gets excellent results."

Kurt: "You know, we had guests in town last week. When Rachel had to reschedule her appointment with him, she acted like she was having a panic attack." (Long pause.) "You don't know any uglier massage therapists, do you?"

Kurt and Rachel went back and forth for six months about the efficacy of Steve's massage skills and the way Kurt felt "concerned" about their working relationship (they actually referred to him as "Ricky" when they argued). Ultimately, Rachel finally relented and found a new therapist—not exactly the outcome I had hoped for or expected. When they visited my office individually, I got to hear their respective sides, and while I occasionally tried to smooth things over for them, I avoided getting involved.

We soon realized that Steve's looks had a lot less to do with Kurt's feelings than the fact that Rachel now depended on someone other than Kurt to feel better. This can be a devastating realization for someone in a relationship that has already been strained by the effects of pain. People in pain often feel immense gratitude toward anyone who helps them find relief, and this in turn can make those close to them suffer jealousy and resentment. It seems to happen a lot, but what's the solution?

Actually, I don't perceive the gratitude as a problem; it is a natural consequence of the pain relief. The problem is the way the partner can experience this gratitude. It is important not to allow unfounded jealousy or other negative feelings to get in the way of opportunities to recover. Conversely, the pain sufferer's gratitude should be tempered with sensitivity toward his partner as well.

Couples need to reach an understanding about

the professionals they rely upon, but arriving at this understanding can often be a huge problem. I see it arise most frequently when one person receives psychological counseling—sharing their most personal secrets and feelings, often about their loved one, with an outsider. While we want to be all things to our loved ones, this is rarely a realistic pursuit. Our personal strengths and limitations make us who we are—the person our partner loves. It is far too easy to become jealous of a person who provides relief to your partner when you cannot. This can happen whether the professional is a massage therapist, psychotherapist, physician, or any specialist who provides a unique service. In general, these feelings are unfounded, but can hinder the ability to feel better, as well as turn a valuable asset in pain recovery into an adversary.

I have found that one of the best ways to avoid this quagmire is to jointly develop relationships with the professionals you rely upon. This does not mean that you should both get treatment from all of the people involved, but it can help to meet them as a couple when that sort of introduction is comfortable and realistic. (In practice, I frequently try to meet patients' spouses so I can learn a little about their home lives and support systems.) In this way you can both learn the specifics of what the practitioner offers, and be more involved in the recovery process. By introducing yourselves together, you will foster confidence in your sense of couplehood. If both of you do this, you can periodically update each other on your progress toward feeling great.

When a joint meeting is not an option, communication is your best tool. You need to discuss in honest terms what specialists are doing for you. If your therapist is beautiful or handsome, that really should not be the most prominent element of your discussions; of course, don't ignore it if that is indeed the case, so there are no surprises such as the one Kurt experienced. Knowing what is happening will go a long way toward putting out emotional fires.

The Joy and Pain of Couplehood

If you are fortunate enough to be in a healthy relationship, you already possess the best resource for feeling relief from pain. Personal support is an absolute prerequisite for recovering a great quality of life. Unfortunately, this support can be compromised easily following the onset of discomfort. The frustration associated with missed opportunities for travel, activities, sexual relations, child care, and much else can be a lot for a relationship to bear. The feelings of helplessness associated with observing a loved one in pain and being unable to do anything about it can change the nature of a relationship in powerful and destructive ways.

It is important to remember a few things:

1. If you are experiencing pain, don't focus on it all of the time. Use some of the tools in this book to help you keep it in perspective. Talk with your partner when there are new things to report, or when you feel there may be opportunities for her to help.

2. If your partner is in pain, try not to make him feel like "damaged goods." It can be easy to treat him like fragile china, but once you do that you change the dynamic of the relationship. He may initially appreciate your efforts, but will eventually resent what he perceives as being patronized. More damaging still is the possibility that he will assume the role of a sick person in response to your behavior. This personality change can be

hard to reverse. Treat your partner with care, respect, and honesty, and treat him as you would if he had no pain at all. This is not to say you or he should be in denial, but you cannot permit pain to dictate the direction of your relationship. Don't give it more attention than it deserves; you both have other things going on that take priority.

3. Be thankful for your partnership. Having someone to communicate with, vent to, and go to sleep and wake up next to is a beautiful gift. Enjoy each other when you can, in ways that remind you of the moments you are not in discomfort. Remind yourselves that pain is transient and should not be allowed to affect who you are as individuals or as a couple.

4. Some people worry that "a little knowledge is a dangerous thing" and that if they learn some of these techniques, they will become their partner's physical therapist. With correct use, most of the methods offered in this book will decrease your partners' dependence upon them or any other form of pain relief. Also, even if neither of you is in pain, they will help you prevent pain and perform better. You might notice that your tennis serve is faster, or your golf drive farther. You may sleep more soundly through the night, or perhaps even be a little less grouchy. (I love the word "grouchy"—it sounds just like what it is!)

Osteopathy
Basics

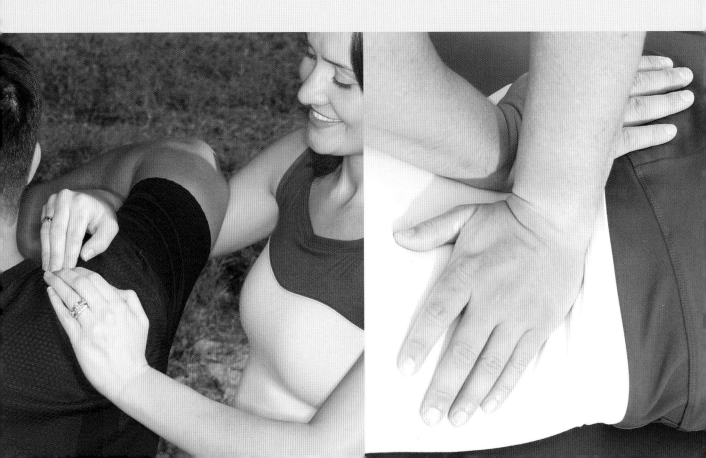

My career path was greatly influenced by some awesomely talented Osteopathic physicians. I truly consider myself lucky to have had the chance to learn from these wonderful people who guided me toward my future. Many of the hands-on applications in this book have their basic roots in Osteopathic Manual Medicine, the treatment modality employed by Osteopathic physicians. While it is somewhat likely that you have encountered and even been treated by a D.O., you may not be aware of what Osteopathy really is. The Osteopathic community has, in many ways, been assimilated into the allopathic (née M.D.) community seamlessly enough that the major differences between the two might no longer be clear.

A physician named Andrew Taylor Still originally conceived of Osteopathic Medicine in the 1800s. Dissatisfied with the medicine practiced by his contemporaries, Still created a system of health care based on the principles that the body has an unparalleled ability to heal itself, and that when it does not, it is frequently because of improper alignment of the skeletal system and the soft tissues surrounding the areas in question. These misalignments came to be known as "Osteopathic lesions" or "somatic"—body-oriented—dysfunctions. I personally shy away from the term "lesion" as many people have come to associate the word only with cancer. The somatic lesion, for most practical purposes is nowhere near as sinister, and is generally a lot easier to treat.

In practice, somatic dysfunctions tend to follow one of two distinct pathways: the viscero-somatic and the somato-visceral reflexes. The viscero-somatic reflex occurs when a problem or pathology of an internal organ (such as the stomach or liver) manifests itself in the musculoskeletal system as a somatic dysfunction. The somato-visceral reflex is exactly the reverse; a lesion in the musculoskeletal system has consequences on the internal organs that are associated with it.

Each area of the musculoskeletal system has a specific set of organs and systems with which it is associated, and these associations are utilized in the art of palpatory diagnosis, where the location and nature of the somatic dysfunction are used to diagnose different conditions. Palpatory diagnosis involves using the hands to feel for irregularities or asymmetry in the musculoskeletal system. By being familiar with the different types of tissue and structural changes that can occur, the physician can begin to utilize this information to come to an accurate diagnosis. Once detected, these lesions can sometimes be corrected through Manual Medicine techniques, in hopes of facilitating resolution of the illness.

To reduce Osteopathy to the most basic terms: You feel around, try to find things that aren't in place, and then gently shove them back where they belong!

Originally conceived as a "complete" system of medical care, Osteopathic Manual Medicine has largely evolved into a complementary method of treatment, often accompanying more "traditional" allopathic treatment modalities. The most popular application of Osteopathic manual treatment is for pain relief; this is the one area where the benefits of Osteopathic manipulation are generally accepted as consistently effective.

There are various styles of Osteopathic manual treatment, and some of them, when not applied correctly, can be dangerous—even fatal. **You will not learn any of those techniques here.** I have distilled the soft-tissue component of my own style of treatment, which I have named Orthokinetic Soft Tissue Optimization or OSTeO™, into these pages. It combines maneuvers based on Osteopathic techniques with elements culled from various other disciplines, including acupuncture, acupressure, shiatsu, dynamic stretching, and other mobilization modalities.

I developed OSTeO for patients who had such acute neck or low back pain that they were unable to turn their heads or bend forward to sit down or pick something up, and were concerned about receiving hard, abrupt spinal corrections. When you look at a dysfunctional segment of the spine, the first thing you need to appreciate is that the relationship between the

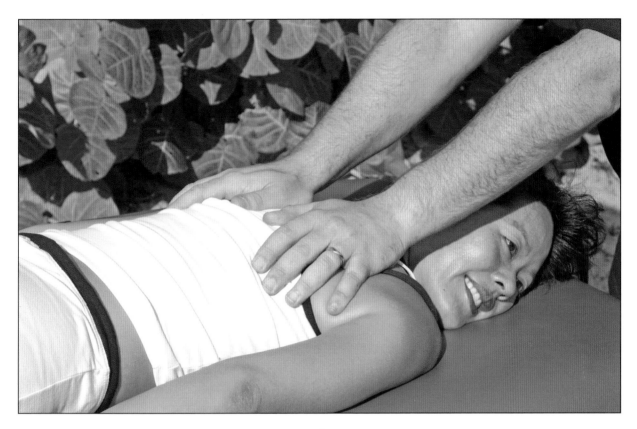

two bones in question is most often out of place by a few millimeters. When I introduce a "thrust" in an effort to correct a cervical Osteopathic lesion, the amount of rotation needed to achieve the correction is most frequently less than 5 degrees—more often closer to 2 or 3. I felt that there had to be a way to effect much of the benefit of the correction without subjecting my patients to a sudden twist or "crack."

OSTeO uses carefully applied, gently pulsing pressure to slowly "urge" a segment back into normal movement. The slow impulses you use will help to decrease spasm and lengthen tight muscles, removing soft-tissue resistance from the treatment equation (muscle spasm and patient resistance are almost always a barrier to effective treatment). This gentle approach will help yield a better, longer-lasting outcome for you and your partner.

You won't learn any bony manipulation techniques or "crunches." Save those for me; if I told you everything, I'd be out of business! In reality, I have selected those techniques that will give you the most bang for your buck, and excluded those that require special knowledge to be performed safely. The techniques in *Back Together* are safe for anyone to apply, and will begin to work rapidly in most cases. I will let you know when you are near structures which could potentially cause you problems, and give you ample opportunity to get far, far away from them.

The Correct Diagnosis

I cannot sufficiently stress the importance of discussing your pain issues with a qualified physician prior to beginning this or any other pain management program. It can be all too easy to assume that your pain is due to strain or stress, but occasionally we find diagnoses that require much more medical intervention than I can legitimately offer here. Certain cancers initially present symptoms of back or joint pain, and can have the opportunity to spread or metastasize if they are not diagnosed in time.

Additionally, much of the hands-on portion of this book is inappropriate for individuals with the following conditions:

1. Cancer, of any type not cured or in remission.

2. Unhealed fracture.

3. Severe osteoporosis.

4. Pregnancy. (I have saved the *pregnancy-safe* techniques for my next book, so if you are thinking about becoming pregnant, hold off a while!)

5. Any musculoskeletal pain syndrome without a clear diagnosis.

For pretty much everyone else on earth, these techniques should be safe and effective. The non-hands-on areas of this book are appropriate for anyone.

The Anatomy and Physiology of Pain

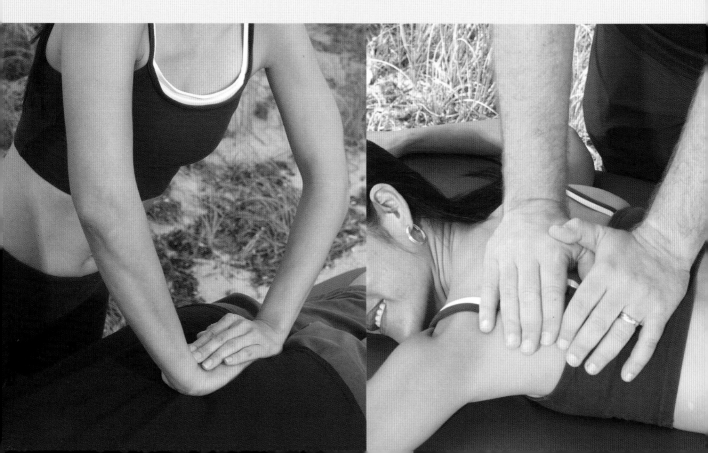

Historically, pain was almost certainly the primary motivator for the creation of what we now call the field of medicine. Today, musculoskeletal pain is an industry unto itself. It is the number one cause of lost workdays. It consumes the highest percentage of all health care dollars spent. If you read newspapers and magazines, you will almost always see someone advertising the "next great thing" for pain. Considering its far-reaching consequences, it seems ironic that its underlying physiologic cause could be so simple and easy to understand.

The medical profession has unfairly burdened some basic scientific principles with what I consider inappropriate degrees of jargon. This is particularly true in Osteopathic medicine, because we have had to spend the better part of our history justifying our existence in an M.D.-dominated landscape. By coming up with lots of scientific names and formulas for the things we could identify through palpation, we proved to the M.D. world that we were "real" doctors and scientists.

Unfortunately, this approach has kept many medical students from learning the fundamentals of this beautiful art form, beyond the elements that are necessary to pass medical board exams. This is especially sad, because in our insurance-mediated medical world, hands-on medicine provides one of the few opportunities for a physician to autonomously act on a patient's behalf without using expensive diagnostic equipment or potentially ineffective or harmful drugs. It is one of the most rewarding aspects of my work; a patient walks into the office in pain, and because of something I do, they leave feeling better.

My office trains medical students, interns, and residents in different aspects of musculoskeletal pain, and I have found that for teaching purposes it has been helpful to develop a paradigm, or model, which reflects the principles I am trying to explain in simple terms and with minimum jargon. Usually, when I pull this information out of the technical tar pit and let students directly observe the results that I achieve in my office, their interest in this aspect of their training is restored.

Virtually all of the well-known authors who have written about back and neck pain have described their ideal model of how musculoskeletal pain evolves. If you have read any of the popular books on the subject, you have probably come across statements such as "All back pain comes from problems with the disc," "Low back pain is actually suppressed stress," or "The pain is caused by a weakness in the surrounding musculature." Someone even went so far as to say that back pain was caused by evil spirits in the spine! In my own humble fashion, let me tell you straight off that they are all wrong, especially the one about the evil spirits. Okay, to some degree they are also all correct as well (except perhaps the one about the evil spirits). Let me explain.

In my practice I have observed that it's a bad idea to try to ascribe one explanation for all musculoskeletal pain. It may sell books or wow an audience, but in the real world, back or neck pain is almost always a combination of numerous intermingled factors. Something causes pain; something else makes it worse; something else prevents it from going away. So any treatment modality that focuses on too narrow a set of parameters regarding an individual's pain is unlikely to completely ameliorate it. The treatment may temporarily relieve the pain, but what have you done to identify and eliminate the underlying cause of the discomfort? How will you keep it from coming back? A person might undergo surgery to fix a herniated disc, but what about the activities or conditions that allowed that disc to become compromised in the first place?

The model I use for musculoskeletal discomfort is what I refer to as the Triad of Pain. Its basic elements are as follows:

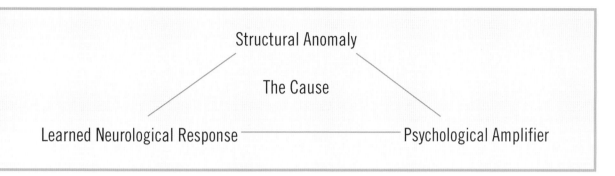

Structural Anomaly

The Cause

Learned Neurological Response ———————— Psychological Amplifier

The Cause

Hovering in the center of the Triad is the cause that activates it. Have you had an injury? Is your chair at work an ergonomic disaster? Are you pushing yourself too hard at the gym? There are innumerable causal events. Your body has an enormous capacity to compensate for activities, movements, or even minor injuries, and the Triad will not usually be activated. It's the activities that stress your body beyond its capacity to compensate that activate the Triad.

Structural Pain

The structural causes of pain are exactly what they sound like: problems with the physical body itself. The problems can usually be identified through physical examination, physical testing, or radiological survey of the area in question. The causes of discomfort can be as subtle as a one-eighth-inch difference

in leg length or as profound as a fractured vertebra. These maladies, when properly diagnosed, generally respond well to treatment. In many cases, the structural causes of pain are a secondary response to an underlying problem such as overuse syndromes (including carpal tunnel syndrome or tendonitis). The primary causes of these secondary response-type maladies can often be addressed through careful ergonomic assessment of the activity involved, and a commensurate change in it.

When a somatic dysfunction is the cause of structural pain, it is most often the result of some causal problem (again, the Cause)—how you sit or stand, the types of exercise you get, or the bed you sleep on, among many others. But if you treat the somatic dysfunction, the structural cause, without addressing the primary cause, the dysfunction will most likely come back.

The Learned Neurological Response

The Learned Neurological Response (LNR) is a relatively new concept in medicine. It came about because we needed to explain why some patients suffered pain long after their injury had been repaired or had sufficient time to heal. It can be difficult to understand at first, so let me try to explain by using an analogy.

When you play a song on a musical instrument for the first time, you know that unless you are some sort of savant you probably won't do a very good job. You play it over and over again, and as you do, you improve until you finally have it down. As long as you continue to play the piece regularly, you will eventually play it well. If you stop playing it, and then play it ten years later, you will probably still play it better than you did the first time. The reason you retain any of your ability is that through repetition, you have established neurological pathways that are conditioned to playing the piece, and have become efficient at it. Once established, these pathways are difficult to eliminate, which is why even after ten years you will still be able to play the piece better than you did at

first. We are designed that way, so that activities which we do routinely require less intellectual effort each time we do them. It is simply a matter of maximized efficiency.

If you extend the analogy of the musical instrument to the injured person, you can see why the pain can continue even after the injury has healed. At the time of the injury, the body established pain pathways that during the healing and rehabilitation process became extremely efficient at experiencing pain. After recovery, the pain can continue for an inordinate period of time because those pathways remain. Breaking them down is one of the processes I will discuss later.

The chronic nature of this type of pain is often frustrating to deal with, and with time provides extra power for what I call "The Psychological Amplifier."

The Psychological Amplifier

In my practice, I see almost every kind of musculoskeletal pain you can imagine, and the variety can be very daunting. However, in spite of the plethora of maladies I have seen, I still broadly group my patients into two distinct categories that are not divined by lab studies, x-rays, or physical exams. The categories are: patients who have an illness, and patients who are ill. Let me explain the difference through the following example.

Lorraine and Stephanie: "Ouch" versus "*Ouch*!"

Fibromyalgia is a poorly understood pain syndrome in which the sufferer experiences pain virtually everywhere. Many physicians who have not really investigated the illness simply write it off, and consider fibromyalgia a "garbage can diagnosis," a label for something we cannot explain and therefore don't really take seriously. If you have fibromyalgia, you *know* that it is real. If you don't have it, be thankful. It is an extraordinarily difficult problem to live with. The reason I chose fibromyalgia for this example is because people who suffer with it are often **miserable**. Their condition can interrupt almost all activity and make tasks such as cleaning the house, or even answering the phone, agonizing. The prognosis for these individuals is largely determined by how they view their condition and the subsequent choices they make. Let's consider two actual patients from my own practice. (Note: I have changed their names.)

Lorraine is a grandmother of four who enjoys nothing more than getting out and spending time with her grandchildren. Her granddaughter, Lori, has Down's syndrome, and as a result Lorraine has become active in many special-needs children's support groups. She travels frequently, and loves shopping and trying new restaurants. If you ask her how she feels, she will almost always tell you she feels great. If you ask her specifically about her pain, she might tell you about how it was tough to fall asleep last night, and how her neck is sore—but even in my office, I need to drag that out of her.

Stephanie is in her early fifties. She is a trained physical therapist, who retired 12 years ago and went on disability. She has been dating the same person for approximately six years because "he can put up with me." She always asks me if I have any patients I can introduce her to so she can dump her current boyfriend. She doesn't try new foods because "I never know how my body will react." When you ask her how she feels, her immediate reply is almost always "terrible," "awful," or occasionally "shitty." What did she do last weekend? "Nothing."

The physical findings of fibromyalgia syndrome are very subtle, but if you listened to these two patients, you would think one had a mild case, and the other had a severe case, but in fact their symptoms are remarkably similar. Let's take a closer look.

In my office I use a detailed subjective analysis of a patient's pain as part of my initial assessment, and to help gauge their progress as we begin treatment. On the scale, 0 means the area is pain-free, and 10 suggests I poured gasoline on the area and lit it on fire. Look at Lorraine and Stephanie's assessments below:

	Lorraine	Stephanie
Neck	6	6
Upper Back	7	6
Lower Back	7	7
Sciatic/Buttocks	4	5
R Anterior Thigh	2	2
L Anterior Thigh	2	2
R Shoulder	6	5
L Shoulder	6	6
R Chest	4	4

I have only included about a quarter of the complete assessment, but the overall similarity between these two patients' subjective evaluations continues. In fact, in several key areas Lorraine's scores are actually *worse* in spite of the fact that she functions better. Incidentally, their physical examinations are remarkably similar, as are their respective past medical histories. They each describe their pain in quantitative terms in a similar way, yet Stephanie is almost completely debilitated while Lorraine continues to have a high quality of life. I often try to book these two patients back to back so my students can see the profound difference between them. It simply boils down to the contrast between *a person who is sick* (Lorraine) and a *sick person* (Stephanie).

As I said earlier, pain can and often does pervade every area of a person's life. How they cope with it emotionally often dictates how their recovery will progress. When illness becomes an integral part of one's personality, it can be nearly impossible to differentiate the sick person from the sickness, and recovery is much more difficult. The Psychological Amplifier is the part of your emotional consciousness that manages how much pain permeates your life in all of its many aspects. The most effective method of controlling the Amplifier is to first become aware of its existence. So congratulations—you've just moved a peg closer to feeling better!

By using the multipronged approach to dealing with pain that I outline in this book, you will have tools to combat structural issues, the Learned Neurological Response, and the Psychological Amplifier.

Living With Pain vs. Just *Living*

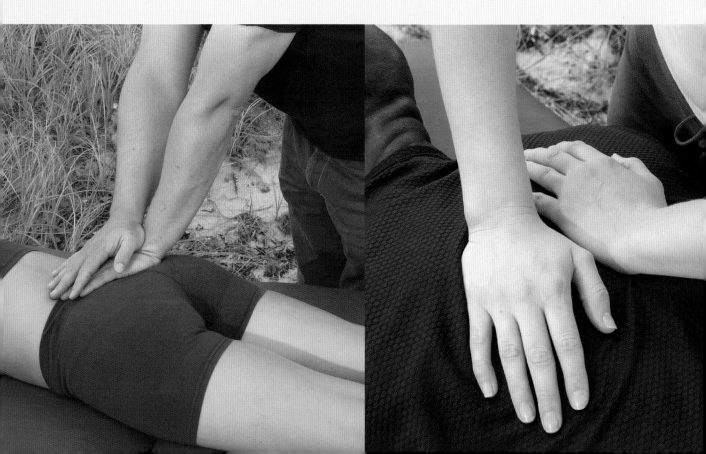

I wrote most of this book in coffee shops. It is amazing how they have become so common—there's probably one across the street from your favorite coffee shop. When I sat with my laptop at my local coffee establishment, I became a magnet for the curious.

"Whatcha doin'?"

"I'm writing a book about back pain." I would reply.

"Oh yeah? I've had back pain for like, forever."

"What have you done to get rid of it?"

"Nothing. I just live with it, I guess."

I could predict that this would be their reply even before they said it, because I had heard it so often before. What I couldn't understand was why they chose to put up with something so unbelievably unpleasant. If a really bad song were playing on your car radio, wouldn't you change the station? If the garbage in your kitchen's trashcan were stinking up your whole house, you would probably take out the garbage, right? I could argue that daily musculoskeletal pain is far more irritating than either of those examples, yet many people choose to "live with it."

As I'm always trying to expand my clientele, I would invariably give these poor souls my card, and urge them to make an appointment. Initially, considering the number of people who took my card, I expected a massive surge in business. The surge never happened. Even people who had heard of me, or who had friends or family members who had come to my office and experienced relief, were unlikely to follow up and get an evaluation. If I ran into them later, they would mumble all kinds of silly excuses.

Why do people choose this path of pain?

Because of the ever-present belief that you can do nothing about back pain—that it is an inevitable consequence of aging, sports, heavy labor, pregnancy, or whatever, and that treatments don't work. The flood of back pain products and books that promise instantaneous and miraculous results invariably propagates this belief. The old adage about things sounding too good to be true holds is certainly the case here. If someone tells you he can fix your back pain but doesn't take the time or effort to understand your lifestyle and anatomical considerations, he is unlikely to achieve any genuine, long-lasting results.

Another concern is the worry that the treatment will be worse than the problem. If you have spoken to enough people who have had various types of back surgery, you have probably heard that the procedure itself as well as the consequent recovery can be quite lengthy and unpleasant. Stories often appear in the news about various medications' newly discovered horrible side effects. Many people are thus leery about the prospect of relying upon surgery or prescription medication to relieve their pain. In fairness to surgeons and drug manufacturers, these options can be the best treatment for the right patient in the right circumstances. However, for the majority of pain sufferers, they are not the most prudent choice.

Learning to "live with it" is not a prudent choice either. There are serious reasons to pursue relief that go beyond the unhappiness caused by the pain itself:

First, keep in mind that if you are involved with someone else, you aren't living with the pain alone; you both live with the pain. When you suffer, your partner suffers and vice versa.

Second, remember that pain is generally an indicator that something is wrong, and by ignoring it or "living with it" you may be passively allowing whatever is amiss to get worse.

Last, pain usually has consequences along what we call "the dynamic chain," meaning that like a domino in a series, your pain may cause you to inadvertently change your body mechanics and favor one side over another, or bear weight on your knees differently, or carry things in your arms in such a manner that your back has to compensate in an unfavorable way. These changes can cause irregular and unpredictable patterns of wear and tear on your joints. What starts as back pain today can result in pain in *many* places later.

While I cannot promise that the concepts and exercises you will learn here will necessarily eliminate your pain, it is likely that they will help. I also know that they are safe, and the consequences of doing nothing are potentially far worse.

Cookies to all of you who have chosen not to simply live with your pain and picked up this book. You will be glad you are here. To those who choose to go through life without taking charge of their discomfort, no cookies for you. (See? Yet another consequence.)

Structural Pain

All structural musculoskeletal pain is in one way or another related to movement. If you experience musculoskeletal pain with a fundamentally structural cause, you can usually find a pain-free position, and as long as you don't move, you can remain comfortable.

Movement is the result of force, the concept you may have studied in Physics 101. How your body feels pain is largely affected by the ways it copes with forces that are created intrinsically (movement initiated from within your body) and extrinsically (everything else—gravity, falling down, etc.).

There are only five structures in the musculoskeletal system that are capable of causing pain at any given location, and each one deals with different specific aspects of force.

1. Muscles create force by contracting, the only thing they can do. They shorten and cause movement through a joint.

2. Joints direct force. The geometric configuration of a joint determines what direction this force can go; for example, an elbow joint can flex in one direction, and shoulders can travel 360 degrees.

3. Ligaments, tendons, and soft tissue put a physiologic limit on the range of motion that force can exert. The stretch reflex activates when muscles are overextended, preventing *intentional* movements that could potentially result in injury. Unfortunately, following an injury, this stretch reflex can "reset" itself to an inappropriate place in a joint's movement, severely limiting one's range of motion. I will talk about this phenomenon later.

4. Nerves initiate force by telling muscles to contract, and then send information about the consequences of muscle-driven force to the brain. (Bend further to pick something up. Quickly drop something that is hot.)

5. Discs and cartilages dissipate all of the extrinsic forces (those not created by the contraction of muscles). They are the body's shock absorbers.

These are the only structures capable of causing pain in the musculoskeletal system under **normal** circumstances. The only exceptions are fractures, myofascial pain, and pain caused by cancer.

If you clinically examine a person experiencing pain, you can almost always trace their symptoms to one of these five structures, irrespective of the complicated names and terminologies that we doctors have ascribed to them. When you have correctly identified the cause, you can go about setting things right. If you have experienced pain, it is likely that you have been given a diagnosis that involves one of these elements. See? Now you know everything you need to know!

Let's look at these structures individually, so we can then create a framework on which to build an understanding of the *structural* mechanism that causes pain, and then address possible methods to alleviate it.

Muscles

Muscles are not actually single structures, but instead are large bundles of fibers called myofibrils. As I stated earlier, the only thing muscles can do is shorten themselves, or contract, when stimulated by the nerve that controls them; or relax. Muscle growth depends upon many factors—exercise, nutrition, use or disuse, and hormonal effects.

In order for exercise to result in muscle growth, the muscle being worked must be taken to the point of exhaustion, just beyond the point where miniscule amounts of damage occur. The body responds to this damage by reinforcing the area in question with a greater number of myofibrils. When this process is repeated over and over, at the gym or through other physical work, muscle growth occurs.

The muscles you exercise are generally referred to as skeletal muscle, and they are the muscles in your body that are under your direct conscious control. (Smooth muscle, as in your colon and cardial muscle in your heart, are under a separate set of neurological controls, and cannot be consciously controlled.) Skeletal muscles are also the most likely to be subject to damage, and subsequently cause pain.

The two most common types of injuries sustained by muscles are strain/sprains and tears.

A sprain/strain injury occurs when a muscle is overstressed beyond the point where muscle growth results. Sprain/strain injuries can take anywhere from days to weeks to resolve. They typically heal themselves, although they can often benefit from restorative treatment such as physical therapy or gradual retraining.

Tears are more problematic, and occur when a muscle is subjected to so much stress that its network of fibers is actually disrupted. In order for a muscle to contract, it must have two points to which it is anchored. In the case of a tear, the connection between the anchors is severed. If it is a partial tear, a proportional amount of that muscle's strength is lost. In the case of a complete disruption, all of the muscle's function is gone, and surgical intervention is frequently necessary, although outcomes following surgery are highly variable.

Muscles are less prone to injury when several factors are met. The most significant ones are:

1. Proper conditioning of muscles appropriate for the activity involved.

2. Proper nutrition. Muscles are constructed largely of protein. If you are involved in a strenuous exercise program designed to increase muscle mass, you need to provide the amino acids (the building blocks of protein) necessary to feed the muscle.

3. Careful stretching and warm-up. During exercise, muscles frequently go into what is known as an anaerobic cycle, where there is inadequate oxygen to serve the immediate needs of the muscles being worked. This causes a build-up of a waste product of muscular activity called lactic acid, and the muscles go into a state of lactic acidosis. You know that this build-up of acid is occurring when you "feel the burn." By warming up, you promote peripheral vascular dilation, which provides oxygen

more efficiently to this tissue and prolongs the effective exercise period before lactic acidosis sets in.

Joints

Several types of joints are found in the structure of the body. We can roughly categorize them as hinge joints (for example the elbow), ball and socket joints (such as the hip), facet joints between the segments in your spine, and sutures, as occur between the bones in the skull.

The more mobile of these joints consist of several structures:

1. The **bones** that establish the basic mechanics of the joint. The way the joints' surfaces interface with each other dictates the direction they can move.

2. The **cartilages** that lubricate and provide shock absorption in the joint by acting as a bearing on which the bones move.

3. The **ligaments** that hold the structures together. Ligaments are like a of group rubber bands that compress structures together, so that the appropriate surfaces of the other anatomical features contact each other.

4. **Bursae**, or fluid filled capsules that act as bearings for the tendons that act around a joint (sort of like a pulley).

5. The **joint capsule**. Some joints, such as knees, are enclosed in a fluid-filled capsule that helps hold the whole package together.

Joints can be subject to many common conditions and injuries. Because they are essentially mechanical devices, they are subject to wear and tear, and these are the types of maladies most likely to affect a joint.

Arthritis is the most common cause of joint pain. The word arthritis is simply a general term meaning inflammation of a joint. It can take many forms, the most common being osteoarthritis.

As joints age, a process of bone destruction and reconstruction constantly takes place. This process is referred to as remodeling. In response to different stressors, bones are constantly trying to reinforce areas that sustain the highest amount of weight bearing, or load. (You have probably heard it said that a bone is stronger after it has been broken. This is because your body figures out that this is a point of high stress, and tries to reinforce it to prevent further injury.) These stresses are especially prevalent at joints, which act as fulcrums across which movement occurs; they are also the areas where bone growth takes place until adulthood. Cells known as osteoclasts, which look a little like Pac Man, move throughout the bony matrix and eat old, stressed-out bone. The counterparts to these osteoclasts are osteoblasts, cells that redistribute new, reinforced bony matrix. (A good way to remember the difference is that osteoblasts, with a B, build bone, and osteoclasts, with a C, look like Pac Man, and chew up and eat old bone.)

As we age, the cartilage that lubricates the surfaces between bones can wear out or become damaged and less efficient at protecting these smooth surfaces. As a result, forces are redistributed in the joint, the continuous remodeling process becomes erratic, and the body forms osteophytes, or little bits of bone that don't really belong there. They tend to spread when not properly addressed. When these osteophytes protrude into the path of joint movement, or impinge upon the pathway of a nerve, the result is pain.

There is one key to dealing with osteoarthritis you must always remember: Disuse of the joints in question will cause the symptoms to worsen. A pianist friend of mine finds that if he even skips a couple of days of playing the piano, it sometimes takes him as long as a week to regain sufficient movement in his fingers. So the underlying motto when dealing with this condition is, as one of my teachers once related, "If you rest, you rust!" When osteoarthritis progresses beyond a certain point, surgical intervention such as arthroscopy, and in extreme cases total joint replacement, are often indicated.

There are other types of arthritis; some, such as rheumatoid arthritis, require careful medical management in order to curtail debilitating long-term effects. Some infectious organisms, such as the one that causes Lyme disease, can cause severe arthritis symptoms. When caught early, these conditions can be managed effectively. Unfortunately, due to their nature, they do not respond well to conservative treatment modalities, and require prompt, aggressive medical intervention.

Joints are also subject to other traumas, the most common being fractures and dislocations. As a general rule, broken bones heal well when they are properly set and given sufficient recovery time. Recovery from dislocations is highly variable; it largely depends upon how much soft tissue damage occurs as a result of the trauma, how rapidly the elements of the joint are "popped" back into place, and whether quality physical therapy is provided shortly thereafter.

Tendons and Ligaments

For purposes of expediency, let's group tendons and ligaments into one group, as the injuries they sustain overlap somewhat, and non-surgical options for treatment of injury to them are very similar. The fundamental difference between these two structures is that while ligaments connect two bony structures, tendons connect muscle to bone. Both structures hold the joints together, and both can be inflamed, strained, or torn.

Ligaments are made of tightly bound groups of fibers that have very little elasticity or "give" relative to other soft tissue structures. They typically hold the bony elements of a joint together. The most common injuries to ligaments are pulls and tears. A pull will usually heal with rest and sometimes with the use of an anti-inflammatory medication. Partial tears will sometimes heal quite nicely when left alone, but complete tears, like muscles, require surgical intervention. As an interesting aside, some ligament repair procedures such as those involving the cruciate ligaments in the knee are enhanced by the use of donor ligaments obtained from cadavers.

Tendons are also created from relatively inflexible fibers, but because they are the transitional tissue between muscles and bones, stress upon them is dissipated by the muscles' ability to contract and relax. They act as cables in the energy transfer system of joints, a critical part of the biological pulleys that allow us to move, augmenting the amounts of force applied to them at their origin. At locations where tendons pass through these pulley systems, they are often lubricated by a surrounding sheath that provides a smooth surface through which to move. Both of these structures can be subject to inflammation, or tendonitis. In the absence of a tear, tendonitis will generally respond to oral anti-inflammatory medications, but in severe cases direct injections of corticosteroids are required. Rest and supportive compression-type sleeves (or even a simple Ace bandage) can facilitate healing, and in mild cases may be the only treatment necessary.

The Central Nervous System

This is perhaps the most important and poorly understood element of the pain model. The central nervous system is responsible for the overall control of the contraction and relaxation of the voluntary muscles. It receives information about proprioception, or the sense of location and movement through space. It also receives information about the malfunctioning of any musculoskeletal system structures, and often informs you of this malfunction through pain. By utilizing a complicated combination of chemical and electrical signals, the central nervous system oversees every aspect of your body's function, and uses systems that you are aware of and consciously control as well as those which function transparently. (Unless you are asthmatic or participate in martial arts, you don't really think about breathing very often, do you?)

With regard to sensation, which is important when you are considering pain, your central nervous system is selective about what it tells you. You are constantly subjected to stimulus from all directions, and your body goes through a complex series of calculations to only make you aware of what you really need to know about right now. Many of these continued sensations are dissipated through a process called accommodation, in which, over a brief period of time, your body slowly suppresses the sensations it does not need. For instance, you don't necessarily want to feel your clothing for long after you put it on. Other stimuli are effectively filtered out by selection (such as the voices in a crowded room, versus the one you are actually trying to hear).

Another part of the central nervous system is fine-tuned to do exactly the opposite. The reticular activating system brings things into your sphere of recognition. If you have ever purchased a new car, you may have noticed cars like yours coming and going a lot more often than you did before. This is not because you suddenly became a style icon and people were emulating your purchases. Your purchase imprinted your new car into your reticular activating system, and made it a more recognizable element in your consciousness. (This system will be very important in our discussion of the Learned Neurological Response later.)

Nerve damage can come from many sources. Trauma can partially disrupt or sever a nerve. Some illnesses can remove the insulation, or myelin, from a nerve, and impede the function of the nerves affected. Other structures can impinge upon a nerve's pathway and interrupt its ability to conduct a signal, as well as cause faulty information (usually in the form of pain) to be sent back to your brain.

Perfectly Engineered

All the talk about what can go wrong with your back may make it easy to forget what an amazing piece of engineering the spine truly is. When you look at its "design," you can begin to truly appreciate the perfection inherent in its form.

At first glance, the vertebrae that make up the spine look similar, simply varying in size. In reality, each region—cervical, thoracic, lumbar, and sacral—is perfectly honed to perform the duties required at that level. For example, the bones in your neck (the cervical spine) are optimized for range of motion and can support movement in all planes, enabling you to rapidly turn your head and focus your attention in any direction.

The lumbar vertebrae at the base of the spine are the largest, corresponding to their need to support a great amount of your total body weight. Consequently, the discs between these vertebrae are also large, and can absorb a substantial amount of shock from activities such as running or jumping. The impact of running, which exerts several hundred pounds of pressure per square inch in some cases, is nearly all dissipated by the time the force reaches your head—which is a good thing, as the force of impact from *walking* would likely cause you a concussion!

The lower vertebrae in the lumbar spine have limited rotational movement, but are extremely adept at flexing and extending, as when you pick up something off the floor. These lumbar vertebrae are supported by a large muscle group that provides tremendous power for lifting, stability, and support.

One of my favorite areas of the spine to study, strictly from an engineering standpoint, is the sacrum. Once believed to be a fused group of bones, the sacrum's tightly bound bones are now known to allow a small degree of movement. The short bands of muscles that attach the sacrum to the pelvic bones and hips provide most of our stability when we walk upright. In fact, the shape of the sacrum itself and the orientation of the pelvic bones to which they it is attached make such walking possible.

In the animal world, the bones of the sacrum extend outwardly to form a tail, which is used primarily for balance and orientation. In humans, the tapering of the bones from the largest at the top, to the smallest, the coccyx (which is buried in dense soft tissue at its end) likely helps dissipate impact as well.

All in all, the spine is an incredible piece of machinery, both a reflection of the complexity of the design and the simplicity of its function. As you approach the hands-on portions of this book, consider some of the functions of the parts of the back you are working with, and you will begin to understand the causes of discomfort; you'll therefore be better equipped to help fix the problem.

So that was a brief overview of the structures that can cause pain. Structure makes up one arm of the Triad of Pain. Now, on to the other two elements of the Triad.

The Learned Neurological Response: Teaching an Old Dog New Tricks

The learned neurological response (LNR) is one of the most complicated aspects of pain, because the storage mechanism your brain uses to retain all of its memories is also responsible for perpetuating the discomfort of chronic pain. How do you overcome that?

If we reflect back to the musical-instrument analogy, the basic mechanism is simple—you practice a piece over and over, and become adept at playing it through the neural pathways you establish. These pathways become so ingrained in your physiology that 10 years later, they still allow you to play a musical piece better than you did the first time.

Patients who have experienced an injury frequently continue to experience pain long after its physiologic cause has resolved, due to the pathways that have been created. These pathways result in irregular body mechanics because of damaged muscle activation patterns. When you perform any activity, your body has preset instructions that automatically engage below the conscious level. Following an injury, the musculoskeletal system alters this pattern to try to compensate for the deficits of the injury. The problem is that your body's normal mechanics developed as you grew from early childhood. The altered mechanics following an injury will frequently change the areas of stress on the musculoskeletal system, resulting in continued pain and *re-injury* of the original site of damage. Other areas closely or even distantly related to that site may also be injured; this cascading effect is known as a dynamic chain injury. Clearly, it is essential to restore the correct patterns of activation and override the pain pathway.

The process of "unlearning" these pathways seems complicated, but it is doable and is based on the concept of neurologic retraining and re-education.

Here is a good example from early in my practice of how this re-education sometimes works:

Stacy is a personal trainer who was involved in a serious car accident. Both of her wrists were broken, and she sustained severe soft tissue injury to her neck and mid- and low back—what we previously referred to as a "sprain and strain" injury. One wrist required a surgical procedure known as an "open reduction/internal fixation," installing pins to hold the fractured bits of bone in place.

Although her fractured wrists seemed to be the most problematic injuries, her wrist pain resolved over the following months. The sprained portions of her spine proved to be the bigger issue. While she lost muscle strength due to lack of use, she never had the opportunity to establish compensatory pathways so her pain activation pattern did not change, or so I had believed.

Her acute back pain improved over a course of months, but only to a point, and when she returned to aerobic dance classes, she severely aggravated the pain. She came to my office exasperated—"How long can this go on? Will I ever work out again?" I had her continue with physical therapy, and prescribed anti-inflammatory medication for several more months. Her next examination was excellent, but when she returned to the fitness club, the pain came back. She felt good most of the time, but when she tried to exercise, she wound up in considerable pain. This was a particularly difficult situation for someone who earns her living as a fitness instructor.

I had Stacy keep a diary of her activities—every-thing she did, and whether or not it caused her pain—from picking up her children at school, to buying groceries, to cleaning her house. I noticed several things when we looked over the list. First of all, even after her injury she was significantly more active than most uninjured people. The second and more important observation was that she performed many activities that roughly replicated the movements and intensity she experienced in her fitness routines but which did not exacerbate her symptoms. For example, picking up bags of groceries out of a shopping cart caused her no difficulty at all, but biceps curls caused her severe pain. Chasing her child around the playground, she was pain-free, while running on a treadmill was excruciating. She agreed that it was strange that similar activities didn't bring equal misery. It seemed that she had quickly restored a normal pattern of muscular activation in the movements she resumed by necessity, such as those involving her children. The activities that she delayed until she felt capable of doing them, specifically exercise, had not resumed their correct patterns. (Stacy is an unusual person in the exercise world. I usually have a really tough time getting patients in fitness professions to allow themselves adequate time to recover. She was actually compliant, and this created frustration for both of us!)

We looked at the various movements that caused her pain and the pain-free movements that replicated them. For example, when she leaned forward to do standing flies, her low back hurt even before she had weights in her hands, while bending forward to pick up her son's toys off the floor was essentially painless. The same basic posture resulted in two different pain states, caused by two distinct muscle activation patterns—one correct and one defective. I had her stand in a straight posture with no flexion and flex forward about 15 degrees, as though she were about to perform her standing flies. I had her do this movement 100 times. By the end, she was getting pretty annoyed.

Imagine how thrilled she was when I asked her to flex 25 degrees and do it in a slow pain-free manner, again 100 times. I loosened up her spine afterwards with some basic soft-tissue techniques, and asked her to return the next day. This time, Stacy went for 35 and 45 degrees. Forty-five degrees had been the range where she experienced pain before

we started this experiment. Now she achieved 45 degrees of flexion, pain-free for the last 30 or so repetitions. I loosened her up again, and I brought her back into the office for the next three days, until she was doing repetitions with her palms on the floor, without pain and with better mobility than before her accident. By re-educating her body to return to its natural activation sequence in pain-free increments, we were able to re-establish pain-free movement.

Unlearning the Learned Neurological Response

If you have been injured, and you continue to experience pain beyond the point where your apparent physical injuries have resolved, you need to consider the possibility that a key component of your pain may be the learned neurological response. How can we apply the example above to your own situation and undo this programmed response? It is simpler than it may appear. It involves five steps:

1. Eliminating or correcting the structural cause of your pain so you can isolate the LNR as the cause

of your discomfort if you haven't already done so (we will get to those procedures later in the book).

2. Identifying the pain-inducing movements.

3. Identifying pain-free or pain-reduced analogs (similar movements to those which cause pain).

4. Reproducing the pain-reduced movements in a gradual, progressively increasing "re-educating" pattern.

5. Gradually reintroducing the pain-causing activities alongside the pain-reduced movements that the individual is already doing during routine activities.

Steps 1 and 2 are easiest. I recommend keeping a diary for Step 2. The pain-free movements will be really straightforward. If you have had chronic pain, they may seem obvious, but I suggest that you actually think about the movements that cause pain. Over time, your body may have become accustomed to a certain degree of pain which you may not be immediately aware of, so think about the actual times you feel pain, and if necessary try to reproduce it in order to see which structures actually hurt.

Identifying the analogous movements that produce lesser degrees of pain can take some time, particularly if you don't spend your life thinking about body mechanics. This is where the diary can really help. Start by keeping a list of your daily activities, and look back at it at the end of each day. Are any of these activities similar to the painful ones? If so, pay particular attention to the pain levels you experience when doing them the following day. Remember, these movements are not necessarily the *same* movements, just *similar*. Also remember that the similarities may not be immediately obvious. For example, bending forward to pick something up off the floor flexes your lumbar spine 90 degrees. Sitting upright in a chair also flexes your spine 90 degrees: totally different physical positions resulting in essentially the same effect on the low back.

After you have identified the reduced-pain movements, you can go about retraining that area to return to its natural, correct activation pattern. First, find a quiet place to work. The movements you are about to perform must be deliberate and accurately reproduced for you to get the necessary effect. Next, make a chart with four columns for each movement you are going to perform. Column 1 has the date. Column 2 should be the number of repetitions you will do. I suggest starting with a low number, such as 10, and building your way up. Column 3 will list the range of motion, in degrees, which you will perform. Column 4 should display your subjective levels of pain, on a scale from 0 to 10, 0 being pain-free, 10 feeling like being burned at the stake! Don't say you have 10 out of 10 back pain unless you really do.

Date	Number of Repetions	Range of Motion	Subjective pain level (0-10)
1/1	3 sets of 10	40 degrees	
1/2	3 sets of 20	45 degrees	
1/3	3 sets of 30	50 degrees	
1/4	3 sets of 40	55 degrees	

When you perform the pain-inducing movement, figure out at what range the pain begins to kick in. Then when you begin doing the repetitions of the pain-reduced movements, start at approximately a third of that amount. If picking up your socks off the floor causes pain at 90 degrees, but leaning over to wash your face at 50 degrees does not, start your repetitions at 30 degrees. If you were to go past 50 degrees washing your face, you would probably start to feel discomfort at some point before 90 degrees.

Perform 10 repetitions of the pain-reduced movement, rest a few minutes, then do it again. After three sets of repetitions, you should return to the movement that causes pain. If possible, do a single repetition of that movement at a slower speed; otherwise, perform it at normal speed. Try to notice if the pain level is as severe. If there is no decrease in the pain level you experience, return to the pain-reduced movement, and perform three more sets of 10. Repeat this process for a total of three complete sets, each time noticing if there is a change in the pain-inducing movements' level of distress. On the first day, most people report a very small but noticeable decrease in pain.

The following day, you may want to try to increase the number of repetitions by a third, and the range of motion of the pain-reduced movement by about 10 percent. At the end of each complete set, do two repetitions of the pain-inducing movement, at a slightly-closer-to-normal speed. (If you are having a tough time following this example, refer to the chart.)

By the third day following this pattern, there is in many cases about a 50 percent decrease in the pain experienced. By the tenth day, the pain level is often decreased by as much as 90 percent or more.

What is going on here is a systematic re-education of the musculoskeletal system. When you follow repetitions of the *pain-reduced* movements with a gradual introduction of the *pain-inducing* movements, you are essentially convincing your body that it can perform these movements without discomfort, and you re-establish a correct activation sequence.

It sounds too simple, and maybe a little silly, but it works. Try it. This process helps knock down another aspect of the Triad of Pain. While each of the approaches you learn in this book may not by itself relieve 100 percent of your pain, the combination of these individual approaches often gets remarkable results. One last note here: If your partner is available to watch you perform your repetitions, she can often help identify areas where you may subconsciously alter movements to make them less painful when you are doing these exercises, and this can decrease their efficacy when you do them in real life. You may unknowingly be shifting your weight, or twisting in anticipation of discomfort whether it is present or not.

A Brief Exercise

Sometimes when I talk to couples about pain, it is not immediately clear to them why a couples-based model is more effective than coming to me, shelling out their co-pay, and having me fix everything for them. It may not be immediately obvious to the pain sufferer why his partner is the best possible resource for his recovery. For the partner not in pain, it may not be clear why she is ideally suited to help her

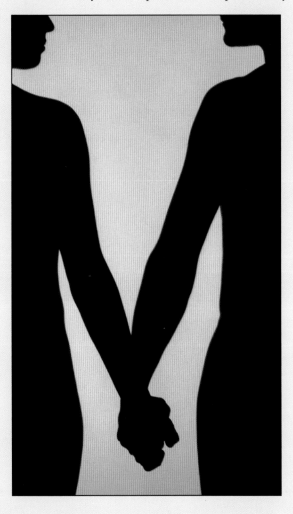

loved one. She isn't a physician—she doesn't know anything about pain, medicine, physical therapy, exercise, or whatever. I offer this little exercise to reaffirm what I am getting at. It's a little bit touchy-feely, but bear with me.

First, I ask them to face each other. Sometimes they both giggle and feel a little silly standing in front of me facing each other, but then I ask them to take a good long look at each other: the face, the body, the whole package, and while they are looking each other over, I encourage them to remember what attracted them to each other in the first place. What traits made you fall in love? Why do you want this person in your life?

After they have thought about this for a while, I ask them to close their eyes, and while still facing each other, take each other by the hands, and experience what their hands feel like. These are the hands of the person they fell in love with—the touch of someone who cares for them more than anyone else on earth. I ask them to really notice what each other's hands feel like, and to remember it. The sensation of holding those hands is profoundly different from holding those of anyone else in the world.

That touch, the feeling it evokes, and all of the chemistry, history, and love it brings up, are what makes it possible for them to help each other heal and perform better in life. I referred earlier to the "joy of couplehood." It may be incredibly difficult to recognize that joy when you are feeling so impaired by pain, but if you try hard, and realize that you are not acting alone in the quest to feel great, you will improve by leaps and bounds.

When I did this exercise at a seminar, I was shocked by how many people approached me afterwards to tell me how much they appreciated it, and how they had not appreciated each other's touch on such a basic level since the time when they first started dating.

Okay, now I'm done being touchy-feely.

Controlling the Psychological Amplifier

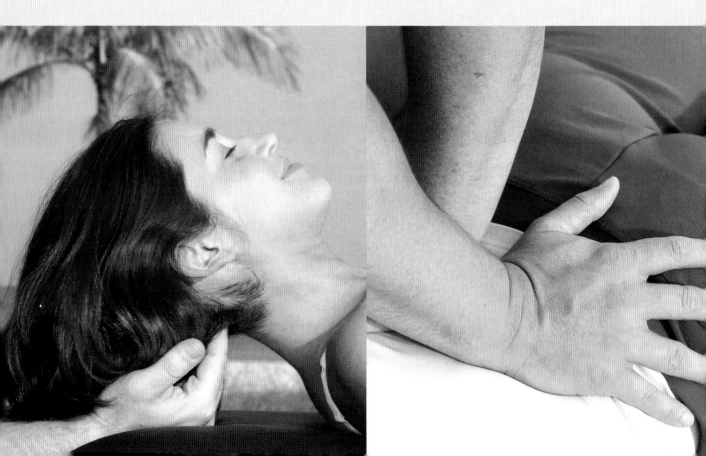

This section was, for me, the most difficult part of this book to write, for two reasons. First, everyone experiences pain in a very personal and internal way. Because of this, trying to supply a single technique for mentally coping with pain is like trying to solve the Middle East conflict with promises of candy and gum. Second, as I began to write this chapter, I was laid up in a hospital bed, receiving intravenous pain medications.

A Good Doctor But a Very, Very Bad Patient

I was seeing patients, and everything was fine, when I suddenly found myself doubled over in what was by far the most excruciating discomfort I had ever experienced. I immediately knew that I had renal calculi—kidney stones, arguably the most painful condition there is (I had actually had them a few times before, but never this severely). I went to the emergency room, where I metamorphosed into that most horrid of beasts, the physician-patient. I knew what my diagnosis was, and even though I had a good understanding of how emergency rooms worked, I demanded pain medication. But the ER staff made it clear that I was not going to receive anything—I was given the customary "shut him up" medicine, Toradol, slightly more helpful with kidney stones than M&Ms—until some basic studies had been performed. (Unfortunately, the current medical-legal situation forces most ER physicians to assume that patients demanding pain medicine are addicts). After what seemed like an eternity, they gave me some narcotics, which promptly took me from a pain level of 11 back down to 2 or 3.

Once I had my wits about me, I realized a few things. First of all, I was now a patient, and not a good one at that. Second, I was not using any of the coping skills I regularly taught my patients for dealing with pain. Remembering to do these things became very difficult during this acute episode of discomfort. Finally, pain made me act like a complete jackass. People cope outwardly with pain in different ways. Some people become quiet and introverted. Others become mean. I became obnoxious, a physician who knew what was wrong with me and whatI needed. Since I wasn't getting it, I was going to torture anyone who came near me until they felt just as lousy as I did.

After receiving the pain medication, I spent the rest of my time in the ER apologizing to everyone I had encountered thus far, and was reassured that it was okay, they understood, given the amount of pain I had just experienced. Then I suddenly had major realizations about pain, how couples experience pain temporally; and about human behavior, which I will share with you now.

Human beings are by and large a compassionate group. If you are fortunate enough to have found someone with whom to share your life (and they have agreed to share it with you—this does not apply if you have them locked in the basement), you have already demonstrated a level of social skill necessary to exist within a couple. One thing which allows us to function as couples is our ability to demonstrate compassion toward the people we care about, and often toward people we don't care about or even know, which explains why the ER staff didn't kick me out for being a jackass!

At the onset of pain, those around the sufferer feel honest compassion for them. Unless there is something wrong with you, you don't like to see people suffer, and you show compassion for someone in pain, even more so if that person is a friend, family member, or significant other. If a loved one is suffering, you may hug them, hold them, and share kind, reassuring words. This, my friends, is the problem. Our natural instinct is to provide positive reinforcement for this negative event—but unfortunately this is frequently the "windup before the crash." Am I telling you to be cold and unfeeling toward your loved one in pain? Of course not! I am saying that this initial outpouring of love sets up the emotional devastation that can occur if the pain continues over time.

The people in the emergency room only had to deal with my lousy attitude for a brief time. If I had stayed there and continued to be difficult, loud, and obnoxious, their patience would have run thin, and eventually, they would want to take turns punching me in the stomach.

Even if you don't become difficult the way I did, the patience of those around you becomes difficult to maintain past a certain point. That point varies with different people, but sooner or later what starts out as compassion for the pain sufferer can turn to frustration when his partner cannot relieve his discomfort and her life begins to be affected by her loved one's pain. This sets up the couple's Psychological Amplifier, and this is why it can be so hard to disrupt.

We can look at the Amplifier as two parts: internal and external. The internal Amplifier occurs in the mind of the sufferer. The external Amplifier results from the dynamic between individuals in a couple. These amplifiers each have their own specific features, and unfortunately, they feed each other unless you are aware of the mechanisms you can employ to break the cycle.

I started to think about the internal component a long time ago, during my first experience with serious pain. The kidney stone episode lasted a total of seven weeks—I needed two surgeries to remove the stones, and to implant a urethral stent to help repair the damage the stones had done on the way out. While at the time this felt like forever, it was temporary.

However, I had what could be termed "chronic" pain for a three-year period, which began during my internship.

I was on my way to the hospital, driving on a major roadway that connects Philadelphia to the outlying suburbs. I was rear-ended at high speed by an 18-wheel semi, which pushed me into the car in front of me, and then squeezed me into the other lane where I was promptly broadsided. After extracting myself from my car by kicking the door open, I went to each of the eleven other cars that were involved in the crash. When I was certain everyone was all right, I fainted by the side of the road.

It was miraculous that I was not severely injured, and at the time, I felt it was truly astounding that I was not experiencing more severe pain as a result of the crash. That was until about three days later.

As the days passed, pain in my low back began to

worsen, to the point where sleep was impossible and activities as basic as walking were extraordinarily difficult. I was limited in the pain medicines I could take because I was seeing patients and could not be impaired. Furthermore, I was one of 16 medical interns, and the others were counting on me for call, rounds, and everything else involved with internship.

The pain affected everything I did, and I was not in a position to take any breaks or use any of the medications that would have helped me to feel better. I was in an internship program where the director of medical education *hated* me and was looking for every opportunity to make my life difficult. I clearly was not to receive any sympathy from the administration.

Thus began a cycle of misery that affected me in every way possible. The pain detracted from my sense of self-worth. My ability to care for patients was impeded. My ability to care for my wife's needs was compromised. My ability to take care of my own physical needs, such as going to the gym, was destroyed. If you suffer from chronic pain, then you have likely dealt with some iteration of these feelings. If you suffer with any sort of chronic pain and you have not experienced any of these feelings, you already have outstanding coping skills, and should probably buy a different book—or better yet write one! My experience with patients tells me that most people have no way of coping with pain emotionally, because most pain we experience while growing up is transient in nature, and largely doesn't effect our emotional makeup.

Something my wife, Donna, once said to me while I suffered with the low back pain from the accident really struck a chord with me, and shaped the way I teach patients to deal with pain. She said, "There are moments you will feel pain, and moments you won't. This happens to be one of the times you do, and it won't last forever."

This was an incredibly insightful thing for her to say, since she had never cared for patients in pain before. You see, the first thing any patient experiencing severe musculoskeletal pain asks me, without exception, is "Will this pain ever go away?" Something about our programming tells us that the pain will last forever. This belief is exacerbated by what I term "The Cousin Murray Pain Paradox" (TCMPP). Almost everyone has the distant cousin or uncle—"My cousin Murray threw his back out like that once, and he was never the same." It's hard to treat patients with TCMPP—if you start out with the prevailing belief that you will never, ever recover, you face an extraordinarily difficult hurdle.

The key to coping with pain is understanding its temporal and transient nature. With a few exceptions, most types of pain can be controlled. Most forms of chronic pain can be reduced if you know how to find patterns. I have always been a fan of Tony Robbins, the personal development guru, and one of his key phrases is "Success leaves clues," meaning that by following successful examples in business, fitness, or whatever, you can learn by example and extrapolate information which may be useful to you. You can use this model for yourself to help break the grip of the Psychological Amplifier.

As you go through your day, even without thinking about it, you have probably identified times when your pain was better or worse than others—the *temporality* of your discomfort. This is the first clue you need to investigate. When do you feel good? Is it in the morning when you first wake up, when you arrive at work, when you are leaving work, or bedtime?

How do you respond to the hiatuses in your discomfort? When in pain it is easy to become mired in a cycle of despair and self-pity. The breaks in your discomfort are your first and best opportunity to begin to beat the Psychological Amplifier.

The Amplifier is, after all, a psychological entity, and as such, must be dealt with by employing psychological tools. One of the most powerful tools available here is positive reinforcement. Earlier, I touched upon the difference between a person who is sick, and a sick person. This is where the distinction becomes important. Somebody wakes up in the morning with a cold, a headache, or back pain. A *person who is sick* says, "I need to do these things today, and oh, by the way, I don't feel so good." The *sick person*, on the other hand, wakes up and says, "I'm sick, and here are all of the things I *can't* do today."

They say if you repeat something over and over enough times, it will become true. Sure enough, the sick person becomes his illness. "I feel awful. I'm so sick. How can I do anything when I feel *sooo* bad?" He says these things to himself, to his family members, and to anyone else who is willing to listen—sitting down for dinner in a restaurant, walking down the street, paying for groceries, wherever.

It becomes the focus of his existence. It becomes his identity. It becomes really annoying!

One of the first steps in breaking the grip of the Psychological Amplifier is eliminating this way of thinking from your repertoire, and perhaps the most effective way to do this is by latching onto those times when you feel less pain. During those episodes, how do you feel? Are you relieved? Are you pissed off because you don't feel that way all of the time? Maybe you don't acknowledge or even recognize those moments at all.

The first thing you should be feeling is **better**. During those moments, appreciate the difference in your level of discomfort, and really think about those ways in which you feel better. Think of the activities and thoughts that brought you to this less painful state. It can be helpful to write notes about the activities that make you feel better, and those that make you worse, as your day goes on. Reading through the notes at the end of the day can help you identify patterns, which can in turn help you reduce your discomfort. When I had my kidney stones and a stent in my kidney, I still needed to go to work and see patients. I still needed to be a husband and father. I probably complained a little more than I should have (okay, maybe more than a little), but

I needed to anchor myself to the moments when I felt a little better in order to help get me through the moments when I didn't. In my case, I felt best when I had just woken up, before I had taxed myself too much physically, and it was this part of the day when I reminded myself that I *did* occasionally feel "not quite as bad," that I was lucky I did not feel worse, and that eventually I would feel better.

When you feel unwell, how do you respond to the question "How are you?" Many people in pain lose their ability to latch onto better, more comfortable moments, and abandon responses such as "Fine" or "Well," and they begin to say things like "Awful" or "Terrible." I could probably write another book about the responses I get to this question. Some of them are funny in a twisted way: "Slightly better than dead," "Take me to the cemetery," "Fine, if you call this fine," or my favorite—"Like week-old Brie." While the responses are funny, the reason for them isn't, but sometimes looking at bad situations from a humorous perspective can help you to get a better grip on them.

Since people, being a polite lot, are always asking you "How are you?," you are conveniently afforded multiple opportunities to change your pattern of thought. You need to change your *mantra,* the thing you repeat over and over again, to change your reality, and to associate that mantra with an internal reflection of the time of the day, or week, or month, when you feel better. "I feel great!"—say it with conviction, say it often, and begin to believe it as you realize that there are moments when you feel pain and moments when you don't.

You might be surprised, but people get really angry when I tell them to do this. Many perceive this approach as lying to one's self, psychobabble—denying the pain exists, and tricking one's self into feeling better. The truth is, your psychological state has as much to do with how you experience the pain as the problem that caused the pain in the first place. You can prove this easily: Think back into your past for a moment. Try to remember an event in your life when you felt really good. Think about the details of that time and what about it made you feel good. If you think long and hard about it, you can almost certainly relive some of the sensations and emotions you experienced, and bring some of those feelings into the present.

An easier example is to think back to an experience that made you very angry. For some reason, we tend to vividly relive the episodes in our lives that aggravated us. We replay them in our heads over and over again, and then we think of what we should have said—the snappy comebacks and responses we could not think of at the time because we were so utterly bent out of shape. You can probably pull up a memory of something that happened in high school, or between you and your parents, or with a boss. When you reflect back to those times, you can feel your muscles tighten up. You may start to grit your teeth. In extreme cases you might even get a headache. Your psychological state influences your physical state in ways you do not even perceive. Your negative emotions have an immediate negative physical effect. Recalling a time when you felt more comfortable will affect your physical pain in the same way. Try it. You might surprise yourself. When you set up a mechanism to shift into an improved psychological state, you implement your central nervous system's ability to bring things into your sphere of recognition. Your reticular activating system, which was previously making you more aware of how bad you were feeling, can be reprogrammed to help you recognize and be more acutely aware of how much better you can feel.

Your Body Remembers All Kinds of Things

I often refer to the notion that your spine is a metaphor for whatever is going on in your life. That is to say, that when your life is going great, you are less likely to experience pain, and when it is going badly, your spine follows suit. Interestingly enough, your spine can also carry with it much more specific manifestations of events that have transpired in your life. Let me share with you an example of this type of "skeletal memory:"

When I was a sophomore medical student, one of my closest friends got engaged. I went to the couple's engagement party and immediately noticed that my friend's fiancée had her head tilted to one side. I asked her about it, and she related that she had woken up with a stiff neck and was in terrible pain. She had scheduled a photographer for the party and was extremely concerned that her photographs would all be ruined by her "crooked head." I immediately sensed the opportunity to become a hero, and told her I could fix her problem. (One of my mentors had just taught me how to deal with this condition, torticolis, a couple of days earlier. I was eager to show off!)

I cleared a space on the floor in their living room, and as her family and friends gathered around, I cracked my knuckles and got to work. After spending close to half an hour, I set up the maneuver that I would use to correct the problem in her neck. I wound up, performed the correction—**crack!**—and knew that I had made her better. I looked down, eager to ask her how she felt, but before I could say a word, she jumped up, ran screaming into the bathroom, and locked the door.

You can imagine how much fun it was having 50 people glaring at me while her little sister screamed "You ruined *everything!*" We crowded around the door, trying to talk her down, and about 20 minutes later she came out, covered in runny mascara. I meekly asked her how she felt. She told me, "Much better." "Did I hurt you?" "No," she replied. At that point I wanted to shake her and ask her what the hell her problem was.

After a while, she explained that at the moment I performed the correction, she immediately relived a horrible experience she had had years before, and it made her scream and cry. This was an example of *somatic memory*, in which a traumatic experience is recorded in the musculoskeletal system. Some physicians suspect that the same neurochemical agents that were released during a traumatic experience can get "stuck" in the area of dysfunction. When the dysfunction is corrected, these chemicals are re-released into the blood stream, and the person relives the experience (according to patients, often quite vividly).

This woman had been carrying the event around unknowingly for years, and when I asked her about it months later, she noted that she had been experiencing neck pain for a long time before it became so acute. She also noted that since I performed the correction, she had been pain free.

Now, Relax: Beating Stress

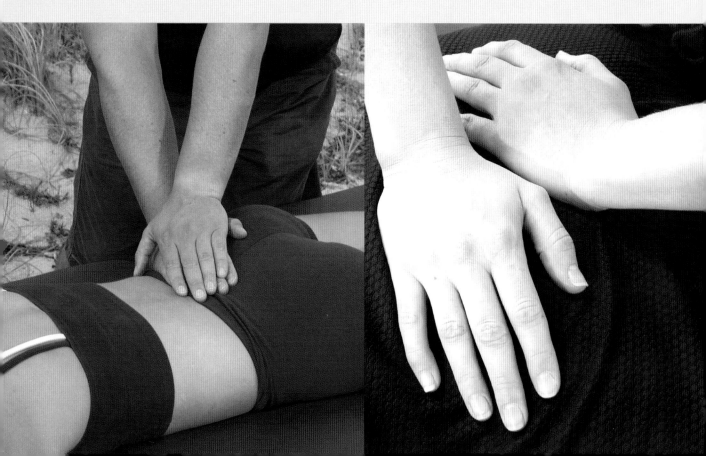

You may have noticed that when you are on vacation, out with friends, or enjoying a good meal, pain doesn't seem to bother you quite as much as it does at other times. Many factors contribute to this. First of all, during those times, you shift the focus of your reticular activating system and your sphere of recognition realigns to notice those things that you enjoy, rather than what causes you discomfort. Secondly, you are distracted from the problems that cause you pain.

Dr. John Sarno, author of *Healing Back Pain: The Mind-Body Connection*, has developed his own approach to back pain. His theory is based upon the belief that most back mpain is a result of sublimated stress, or what he calls "tension myositis syndrome." His approach is extremely successful because it focuses on the psychological facet of the Triad of Pain, which most practitioners tend to overlook. We can easily demonstrate that stress can amplify the effects of pain, and that relaxation helps to relieve it, by looking at examples in daily life. As I mentioned above, simple pleasures such as travel and leisure activities often reduce the effects of pain. Sometimes something as small as dessert can distract us from pain and provide us with enough comfort that the pain "goes away," however briefly. On the other hand, when things go badly at work, or school, or in our relationships, we quickly notice the pain worsening as though someone were turning up the volume knob on our discomfort.

There are plenty of ways to relax, and it is critical to your recovery that you identify easy ways to achieve a peaceful, relaxed state. Look at events in your own life. You may need to make another diary. What activities cause you to feel more relaxed and rested?

Some people turn to yoga or cardiovascular exercise as an outlet for their stress. How about a good book? The key here is to set aside time to do these things on a regular basis. I know from personal experience that if I let more than two days pass without going to the gym, I become cranky, my sleep suffers, and before too long I become a serious mess. Find your outlet, and work with it.

Creativity As Therapy

Pain often makes people forget the positive aspects of their lives. Hobbies or artistic diversions can help restore a sense of normalcy. Giving "birth" to one's own creations often provides a sense of satisfaction which can all too often be absent from the life of a pain sufferer.

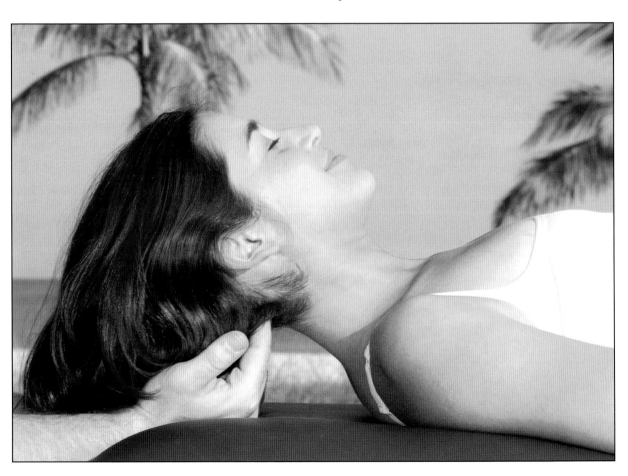

A patient of mine has severe degenerative disc disease, which used to cause him excruciating low back pain. One of the first things he did when the pain really began to get out of hand was to stop playing the piano. When we started to work on his back pain, we talked about his life in general, and the things he liked to do. He related that up until six months before he had been playing the piano as much as 2 hours a day, but when the pain got out of hand, he simply stopped. I needed about a week to gather his x-rays and MRIs to put together a treatment plan, but one of my first recommendations was to start playing the piano again.

When he returned to my office the following week, he was in a much better mood; the resumption of piano playing had given him back a part of his life—a creative outlet—that he had neglected for months. Remember, someone who feels better perceives discomfort very differently from someone who is miserable. Friends have told me that activities as varied as writing poetry or short stories, painting, or even singing in the shower can help bring them into a more relaxed and comfortable state.

My Partner is in Pain

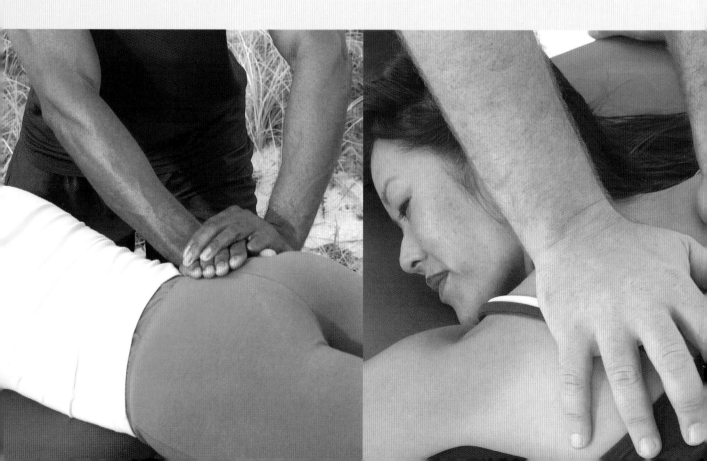

Emotionally, loving someone in pain is often as difficult as experiencing your own pain. It is hard enough to endure witnessing the suffering of your significant other, but the ramifications go much further than that. Household chores, childcare, earning income, even the quality and frequency of sexual intimacy can all be compromised by pain. The two of you may be unable to participate in the regular activities of daily life. Compassion can easily turn to frustration and resentment, feelings that are neither constructive nor helpful, and will eventually cause your partner to feel even worse. Many individuals feel as though the situation is not what they signed up for.

I take care of a couple. The husband fell off a ladder at work about three years ago, and their lives were affected in every way imaginable. He was unable to work. He could not lift anything heavy. His sleep was horrible. He could not travel in the car for more than 20 minutes without experiencing severe pain. One day his wife came in for an office visit and we began to talk. "He is driving me crazy," she said. "He won't get any better. He won't follow through with his exercises and he doesn't take his medications the way he's supposed to. He is just driving me crazy." (Incidentally, when dealing with couples, I try to obtain permission from both members to share information pertaining to their treatment when they seek out individual *Back Together* counseling.)

We discussed it further, and decided to take this to the next investigative level. I brought them into the office together and asked them in-depth questions about what was actually going on. It turned out that not only was he doing the exercises he was supposed to be doing, and taking his medications as ordered; he was actually doing *more!* He had joined a gym and had already lost more than 25 pounds. He was working part time and his new job left him sore at the end of each day, so perhaps he was complaining more than he might have otherwise. She had fallen into the classic trap that catches many partners of pain sufferers: She resented the way his injury was affecting their life, blamed him for the way he felt, and could not recognize his efforts to feel better.

Her resentment regarding the previous three years, combined with some additional complaining on his part, rendered her unable to see that he was actually doing great! When you feel resentment and assign blame, you become unable to support the one you love in any meaningful way. This unconscious distortion is common in situations like this, and it is critical to remember that it is unconscious; she was not doing it on purpose any more than he was deliberately experiencing pain.

If you ask the average person how they can help their partner in pain, they will almost always tell you, "Be supportive." That, ladies and gentlemen, is the biggest piece of BS advice I have ever heard.

What does "Be supportive" really mean? Everybody says it. Should you pat your partner on the back several times a day and say, "There, there" or "Your doin' just fine" or "Hang in there"? Being patronizing is rarely helpful, and when someone feels lousy, there is no positive way to respond to "supportive" comments like these.

The most effective form of support is to first recognize that the one suffering is not doing it because they want to. They aren't trying to ruin your day, and it's not their fault. Second, you need to open a dialog with them to establish what your respective needs are. A pain sufferer will frequently concentrate her depleted resources on areas of home life that she thinks are important to her partner, when in fact his needs or desires are completely different. What aspects of his life are affected the most? Which aspects mean the most to him? Are there ways in which she can honestly improve those areas without making her pain worse? If she has the capability to do 17 things in a day, and he is asking for 18, are there a few they could compromise on to help make things better?

Next, he needs to help reinforce the positive triggers that she is trying to cultivate. They can both determine the best times her day and take advantage of them. They can do more activities together as a couple when she is able, and reincorporate activities that may have been lost, in order to restore a sense of normalcy. He will feel better doing the things he wants to do with her, and she will respond to the positive reinforcement she observes, along with the sense of well being she can achieve by participating in "regular" activities. This too will help provide additional emotional triggers that will bring her into a better psychological state.

Sex: Feeling Really Good Is Good for Both of You

Unfortunately, sexual intimacy is one of the first things that go by the wayside when pain occurs. This is truly unfortunate because there are so many things that are therapeutic about intercourse. From a purely structural point of view, sex mobilizes spinal segments in a slow rhythmic fashion, which is often quite helpful. The endorphin release that occurs shortly before and during orgasm provides natural pain relief that can last for hours following lovemaking. Additionally, the closeness of intimacy positively influences the psychological ramifications of pain on the relationship for both partners. The one not in

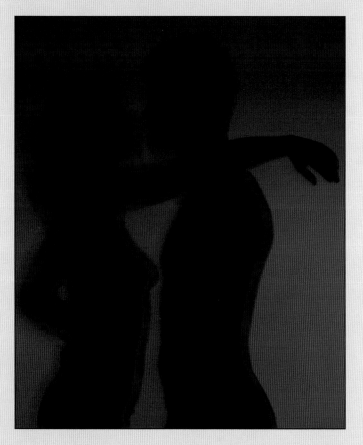

pain will feel closer to his partner. The partner in pain, who may have felt alienated by the omnipresent condition, will feel drawn back into their world. Like I said before, a loving partner is the best resource for relieving pain.

Now I should make it clear that in many instances, your paradigm for lovemaking may require a makeover. First, a pain-free or pain-reduced position needs to be identified. The more active partner may need to take the reins more than either of them is accustomed to in order for both partners to feel satisfaction. Also, sexual intimacy may not necessarily mean traditional intercourse. Oral and manual stimulation can provide most of the positive benefits I already mentioned, with minimal physiologic risk. A pleasant outcome for both partners may require some trial and error before you can achieve success, but it will be well worth the effort!

One further note. If intimacy has been abandoned due to pain, its slow reintroduction may hit some roadblocks before a comfortable zone can be identified. This is absolutely an area where patience is critical. When sexual expectations are high and you don't achieve the desired outcome, frustration can set in, opening a whole emotional Pandora's box. Begin the reintroduction with a clear understanding that there are obstacles to conquer, and that success is not guaranteed from the get-go.

Introduction to the Hands-On Techniques

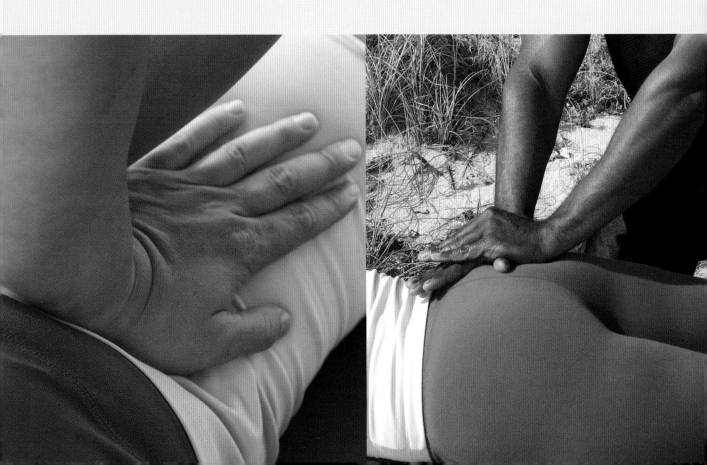

I spent a long time figuring out how to present these techniques in a way that would be immediately beneficial. It's difficult. When couples come into my office, I generally show them methods that apply specifically to them. Here, I want to present a general approach to many types of pain, so I have selected those techniques that I believe will offer you the most "bang for your buck."

Little Things and Their big Effects

A story:

An automobile auction brought exotic cars to our city from all around the world, and because of the value of some of the vehicles, many of the higher bidders brought along their own personal mechanics to help sort out their purchases. The highlight of the show was a well-maintained Ferrari 250 GTO with a complete service history and historic race provenance. The auctioneers hoped the car would sell for approximately $500,000, but the bidding ended at over a million dollars!

The vehicle was moved over to an inspection area, where mechanics working with other bidders had already congregated to admire it. The new owner fired it up, but instead of hearing the melodious roar that only an Italian car can produce, what he got was closer to "Chitty Chitty Bang Bang." The mechanics had a variety of theories about what was wrong: "It needs a new ignition." "Its valves are shot." The car obviously needed thousands of dollars of work to run properly, and the new owner was none too happy.

After an hour or so, an Italian man about

85 years old was escorted over to the inspection area. He did not speak a word of English, but it was explained that hewas an expert on Ferraris. He leaned over the engine and as his escort revved it a couple of times, he listened to various areas of interest. He gave a knowing nod, reached into his pocket and produced a penny. Using it as a screwdriver, he adjusted something on one of the carburetors that resulted in the glorious sound everyone expected. He nodded again and walked away.

The moral of this story is that little things can make a tremendous difference, and while some of the techniques you are about to learn may appear to be minuscule, you can be sure that they can all have a profound effect on how you or your partner perceive pain. I know what you are thinking: "That old man was an expert—of course he knew what to do!" Yes, he was. It is my hope that when you finish this book, you and your partner will be experts too.

Because the little things *do* matter, let me lay down some ground rules before you try the techniques.

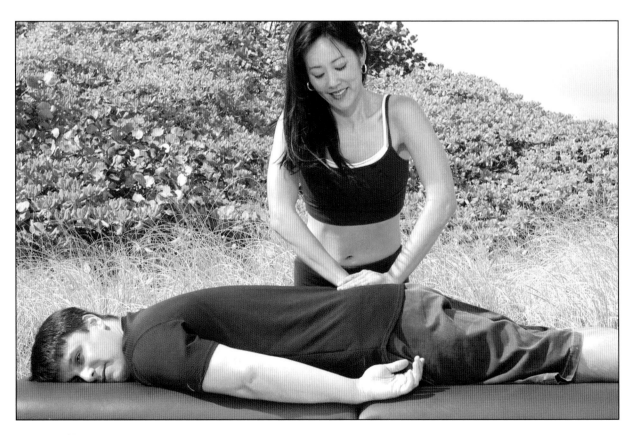

The Ground Rules

1. Unless you are specifically instructed to, **never** apply pressure directly to the bones that make up the spine, *especially* the spinous processes (the central row of little bumps that run down the length of your spine).

2. If the technique causes extreme discomfort, **stop**. These techniques should, by and large, be comfortable and relaxing for the person receiving them.

3. Do not perform these techniques on an acute injury. Acute injuries require assessment by a qualified physician prior to any manual treatment.

4. You may occasionally feel a "crack" or "pop" while applying a technique. These sounds are not dangerous and should not be cause for concern by themselves. Conversely, this "crack" should not be a goal in your treatment. When patients come into my office feeling they need to be "cracked," they sometimes feel they have been ripped off if they don't hear a big loud pop during the treatment. The techniques you will learn in this book are not intended to manipulate joints or bony structures; those maneuvers need to be applied by a trained physician in order to be safe and effective.

5. I have gone to tremendous lengths to ensure that these techniques are safe for almost everyone. However, **please consult your family physician prior to beginning this program.** Certain techniques are not appropriate for certain conditions, particularly with patients who have undergone orthopedic surgeries.

6. Pregnant women should not have pressure applied to their backs while lying on their abdomens after the first trimester of pregnancy. Certain sacral maneuvers are known to induce contractions.

7. Individuals with cancer not in remission should not have these techniques done to them.

8. Always familiarize yourself with your partner's anatomy before you begin work. Even if you have performed a given technique a thousand times, palpate your partner's spine before you begin to apply the technique again. You may be surprised by what you find.

9. Be sure to communicate with your partner continuously. Do not fall into a rut where you believe you know what your partner needs before you even begin. Always discuss each other's needs.

10. When you are done performing a technique, discuss the outcome. This is the most effective method to ensure that every time you try to help each other, you will improve and hone your skills. You can get feedback about which techniques are most effective, as well as about how you can improve the application of any one of them.

11. Experiment with different techniques, as well as how often and in what order you apply them. It may take some time to establish specific protocols that are perfect for your individual situation.

12. Most importantly, enjoy yourselves.

Remember to Breathe

The oxygen you breathe in is the most fundamental element you require in order to function and survive. Unfortunately, I often see pain sufferers demonstrate an altered breathing pattern. Breaths become shallow and inefficient. One way to immediately affect how you feel is to establish a high-quality breathing pattern, one that effectively oxygenates the lungs and allows your tissue to feel strong and healthy.

Each day, set aside time to take slow deep breaths. Allow the air to expand your lungs by consciously feeling your chest go up with inhalation and down with exhalation. In addition to allowing for more effectively oxygenated tissue, the deep breaths have another effect; your cells dispose of certain waste products through your lymphatic drainage system (a tightly packed network of tubes linked by "nodes" of lymph tissue which extract infectious agents and waste from your body). The main collection site of this network is the *thoracic duct*, which disposes of all of the waste products. This duct is stimulated and "pumped" by deep breaths, facilitating effective lymphatic drainage.

For your breathing routine, try to stand in a comfortable position, with your feet slightly farther apart than your shoulder width. Take a deep breath, feeling your diaphragm pulling down toward your center of gravity. Continue to take in air until you feel you have reached maximum capacity. Hold your breath for a few moments (five seconds or so), and then let it slowly escape, gently forcing it from your lungs. Feel your ribs lower and the volume of your breath decrease. When you feel you have gotten to the end of the exhalation, force out a quick, hard breath, and then repeat the process. You should try to take 10 deep breaths several times each day. You will be amazed at the impact this simple activity will have upon your sense of relaxation and your overall energy level.

The reason I mention this point now is that all of the hands-on techniques described in this book are aided by good breathing. When you are performing these techniques on your partner, remember to encourage him to breathe properly. In addition to the points mentioned above, breathing facilitates movement of almost all of the vertebrae in your spine, and mobilization is your friend when addressing the mechanical aspects of pain.

The Basic Moves

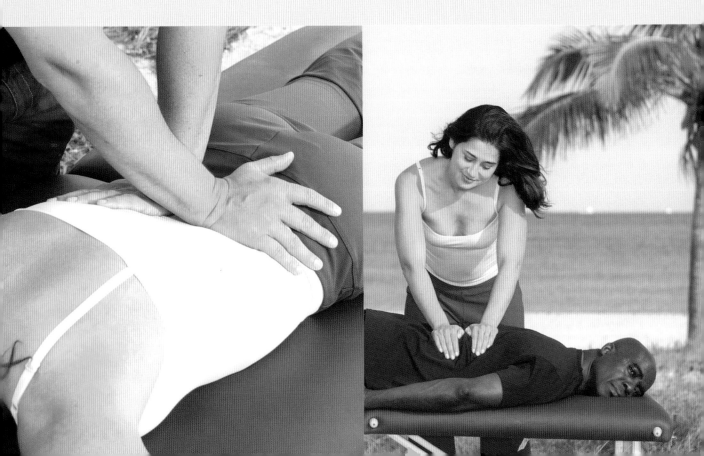

Orthokinetic Soft Tissue Optimization, OSTeO, requires that pressure be applied in a very specific manner. Unless otherwise specified, the pressure your hand applies when utilizing these techniques *should be distributed evenly throughout the palm*. The pressure needs to be firm—you are working through several layers of tissue. Occasionally, you will be instructed to apply pressure with the tips of your fingers.

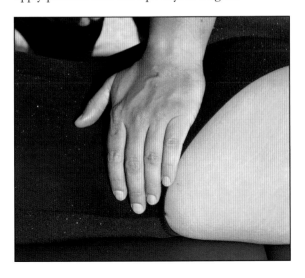

When you first apply pressure, for example to the lower back, start by resting your palm on bare skin if possible, just lateral to (to the side of) the spine—**not** on the bones of the spine itself!—with your fingers pointing away from the spine (see photo left). Slowly increase the pressure and try to feel the layer of fat just below the skin being compressed (it doesn't matter how much you work out, *everyone* has this layer of fat). You should feel muscle just beneath that. As soon as you feel the barrier between the fat and the muscle, stop. Your hand will now be applying pressure at the depth of the first layer of connective tissue, or subcutaneous fascia. Next, while maintaining this level of pressure, pull the layers you are compressing gently away from the spine, using your palm and without sliding on the skin, until you feel the tissue pulling in the opposite direction. This is the first barrier of resistance, one of two you are trying to affect using this treatment style.

If you continue to apply this gentle traction on the skin, with slow even pressure, and without hurting your partner, you will notice an interesting thing: The distance between your hand and the spine will slowly increase as the myofascial layer relaxes. This is the basic principle of myofascial release, and you will be shown places where this type of release is useful in relieving pain.

The next barrier of resistance you will want to affect comes at a deeper layer. Without removing your hands from your partner, release the traction you are applying to the myofascial layer, and relax the tension back to the surface where your hands started. Now increase the pressure downward until you are squeezing the muscle; it will feel thicker and more resistant to pressure than the fat just on top of it. As you increase the pressure, you will see the spine start to bend slightly in response. This is as hard as you need to press. Now, press and relax, alternating at approximately twice the rate of your partner's respiration. As you repeat the cycle of pressure and relaxation, you will soon feel the muscles relax, and the amount of pressure you need to apply to get the spine moving will decrease. All the moves relax the muscle alongside the spine, and introduce basic mobilization to the vertebrae, or spinal segments, associated with those muscles.

The lower back is a terrific place to learn how to apply these two types of pressure and gauge the response, since the muscle groups are relatively large, easy to palpate, and difficult to harm. As you grow accustomed to the sensations you are feeling for, you will have an idea of how to apply these techniques to other areas of the body.

There are a few other things to be aware of before we actually look at the techniques themselves. First, non-acute sources of pain often respond well to heat, and conveniently, your hand supplies it; simply resting your palm on a painful area can be therapeutic by itself. Second, the length of time needed to achieve relaxation or release can vary from seconds to several minutes, so don't rush. Last, I will refer to directions of force in some of the descriptions. Please look at the diagrams on the next page to familiarize yourself with the terms before you even look at the techniques.

On the pages describing the techniques, you will see special "how-to" photos marked with green hands, arrows, and/or circles. The hands indicate hand placement. The circles indicate where to apply pressure. The arrows show the direction in which to apply force. You will also see red lines running down the spine, to remind you to avoid touching the spine. As I said in the ground rules, never apply pressure directly to the bones that make up the spine, *especially* the spinous processes (the central row of little bumps that run down the length of your spine).

It is easy enough to figure out what the causes of pain are, but ultimately, that's not why you got this book, is it? How do you make the pain go away? How do you stop it from coming in the first place? Once you get rid of the pain, how will you keep it from coming back? If you have ever woken up with a stiff neck, you know that at that moment you would do *anything* to feel better—you don't care what the cause is! If you have been walking around with chronic pain, by now you have probably tried loads of things to make it go away. Now's your chance to get rid of pain.

Onward to the techniques!

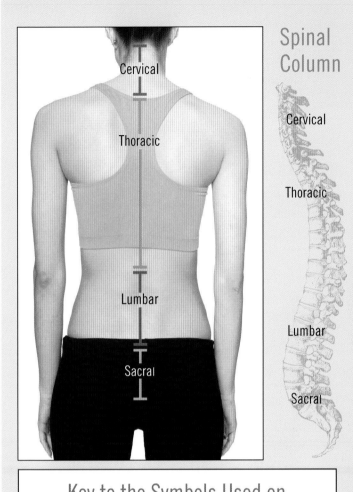

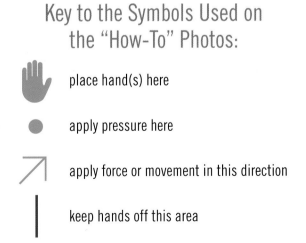

Key to the Symbols Used on the "How-To" Photos:

place hand(s) here

apply pressure here

apply force or movement in this direction

keep hands off this area

Frontalis Release

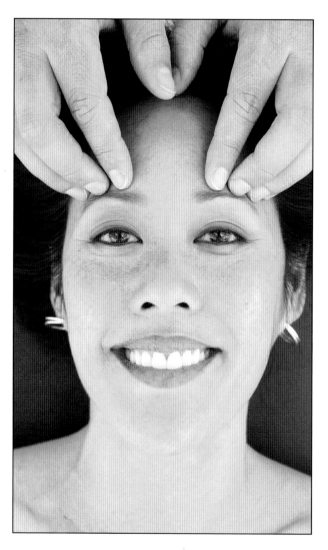

What the Technique Does

Useful for reducing headache discomfort and tension.

Why It Works

This technique releases tension in the frontalis and corrugator muscles, as well as their associated soft tissue directly above and between the eyes.

How It Is Done

I love this technique because of its innate simplicity and the great results it can provide. Begin by asking your partner to lie on her back. Place your fingers across the ridge of bone lying just underneath the eyebrows, with your index fingers meeting right on the center line of her eyebrow. Draw the skin you are pressing underneath your fingers with slow gentle tension in a circular pattern, first with your fingers going toward each other, then traveling away from each other. Begin with small circles and gradually increase in circumference as you feel the tissue start to relax. Your partner should be relaxed, taking slow deep breaths with her eyes open and gazing straight ahead.

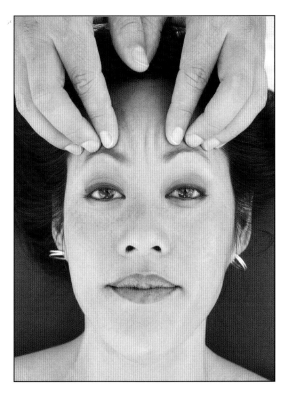

Variation

After you have completed this technique, leave your fingers in the same location on your partner's face, and gently draw the skin toward the top of her head until you begin to feel the tissue beneath the skin resist the traction. Hold the skin with the tension continuing in this same direction until you feel the tissue release. Then reverse the direction of the traction down toward her face, again waiting for the resistance to disappear.

Hint

Combine this technique with the Supra-Maxillary and Cervical Releases (Techniques 2 and 4) to equip yourself with an extremely powerful headache-relieving regimen.

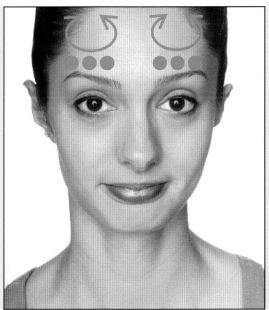

Supra-Maxillary Release

What the Technique Does

Diminishes sinus pressure and pain, reduces headache discomfort.

Why It Works

By relaxing the soft tissue crossing under the zygomatic arch (the cheekbone), you stimulate a reflex point which can diminish pain and pressure in the maxillary sinuses.

How It Is Done

Locate the groove in the middle of the cheekbone beside and slightly below the bottom of the nose. Begin by applying soft pressure in a direction straight through your partner's face toward the table or surface she is resting on. Once you feel the soft tissue resistance build

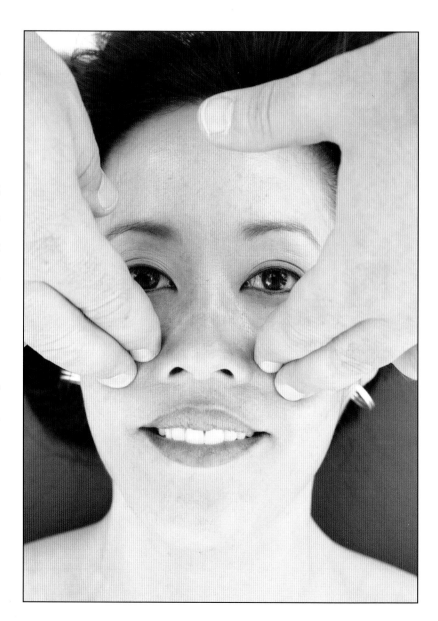

up to the level just before you are pressing against bone, rotate your fingers in a circular pattern, with a diameter about the width of a pea. Go for several minutes in both directions. Your partner may report that she feels as though her nose is running.

Hint

It is important to note that this area might be tender if your partner is experiencing a sinus infection or migraine headache. In this case, apply lighter pressure and gradually increase as tolerated.

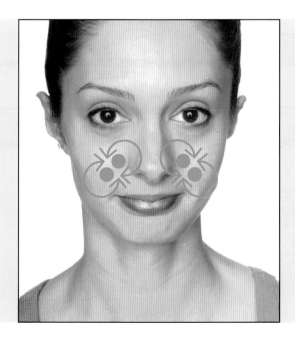

Suboccipital Release

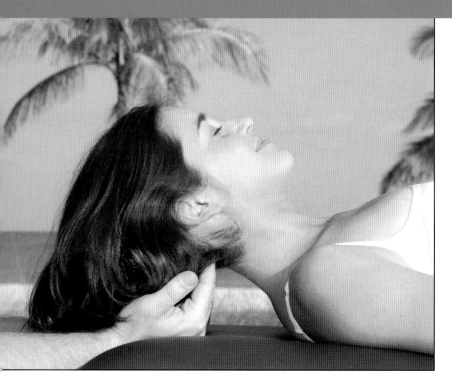

What the Technique Does

Helps to reduce neck stiffness and pain and relieves sinus pain and pressure.

Why It Works

There is a small ligamentous band of tissue between the first cervical vertebrae (the atlas) and the bone at the base of the skull (the occipital bone). The occipital nerve passes through this band of tissue. When under tension, this nerve can cause headaches and in extreme cases nausea and dizziness. This area seems to be a focus of tension and stress for many people, and relaxation of this tissue can be extremely beneficial.

How It Is Done

Slide your fingers up your partner's neck until you locate the very base of the skull (you will know it by the bony ridge which protrudes from the back of the skull.) Now, move your fingers into the area of soft tissue right below that ridge. Using the palm of your hand, gently lift your partner's head off the table and extend your fingers so that they support the weight of her head, and her head is suspended over your hands. As she relaxes, her head will slowly sink into your hands. When it is in the palm of your hands, repeat the technique once or twice to ensure total relaxation of the area.

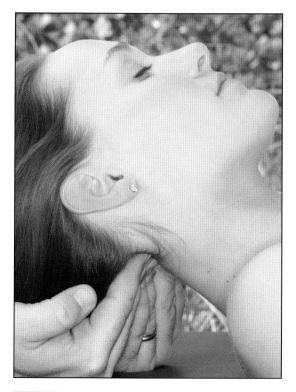

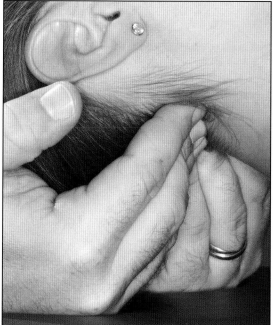

Hint

It is extremely important that your partner not try to press her head into your hands. Ask her to try to relax all of the muscles in her neck and allow gravity to draw her head down.

Variation

You can perform this same technique between each of the cervical vertebrae, relaxing each segment in order from top to bottom. Be careful not to apply pressure to the vertebrae themselves; work on either side of them. As you progress down the cervical spine, you will no longer be able to suspend your partner's head over your hands. At this point, apply pressure with your fingers until you feel the tension release. It may take some practice to feel this subtle change, but you can rely upon communication with each other to help.

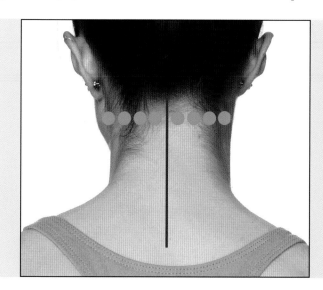

General Cervical Release

What the Technique Does

A nice complement to the suboccipital release, this simple technique reduces neck stiffness and discomfort.

Why It Works

There are multiple muscles running through the posterior neck (back of the neck), including the rectus, semispinalis, splenius, and longissmus capitis muscles. This technique addresses these muscles as a general group instead of one at a time.

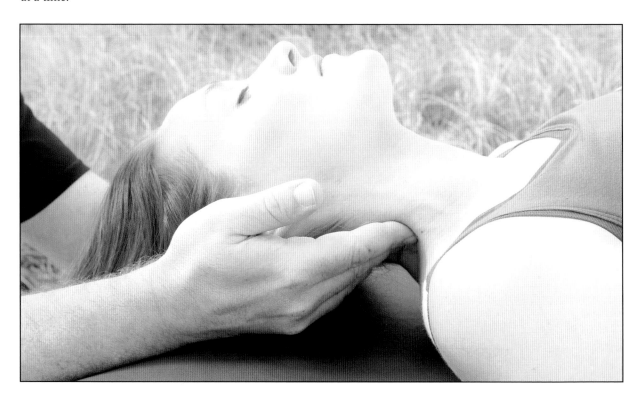

How It Is Done

Line up the fingers of both hands along the sides of your partner's neck, applying gentle, even pressure through your fingers. Using a slow circular motion, apply "waves" of pressure, beginning at the base of the neck and ending just below the occipital bone at the base of the skull. Again, remember that your fingers do not slide along the surface of the skin; they "drag" it in the direction of the tension. You should reverse the direction of the wave in order to achieve relaxation of the fascia in both directions.

Hint

Only apply pressure to the posterior portion of the neck. The carotid arteries travel beneath the surface of the skin on the side of the neck, and aggressive pressure to this area can result in dizziness and worse if your partner has any atherosclerosis (hardening of the arteries.)

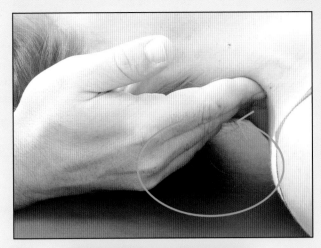

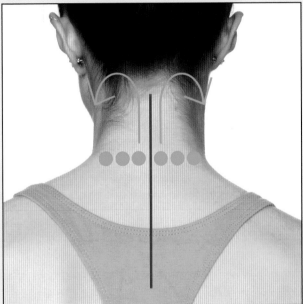

Seated Trapezius Release

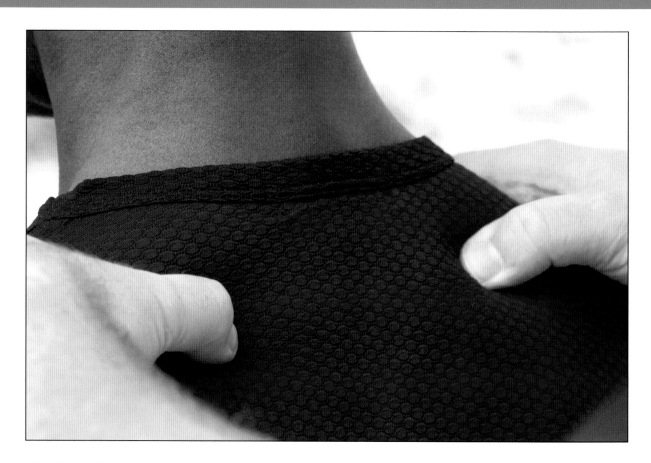

What the Technique Does

Reduces shoulder and lower neck pain and stiffness, such as can result from prolonged computer use or driving.

Why It Works

The postures involved in driving, typing, computer mouse use, or any other activity which forces us into a seated

position with our hands outstretched in front of us for long periods of time causes extreme stress to the support muscles of the neck and shoulders. The trapezius, the large triangular muscle on the back of the shoulder, carries much of the burden of this stress. This technique relaxes the most stressed portion of this muscle.

How It Is Done

Place your hands on your partner's shoulders, with your thumbs on the back, and your fingers on the front. Use your thumbs to locate the thick "belly" of this muscle. Your partner may tell you exactly when you get to this spot, as it may be quite tender. When you have identified it, apply gentle, slowly increasing pressure in a small circular pattern, changing directions periodically, until you feel that point "dissolve" beneath your thumbs.

Hint

At the end of a long day of driving, combine this technique with the Prone Trapezius/ Rib Release (next) to help avoid problems the next day.

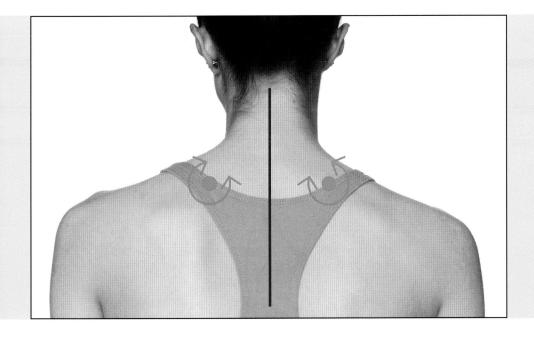

Prone Trapezius/Rib Release

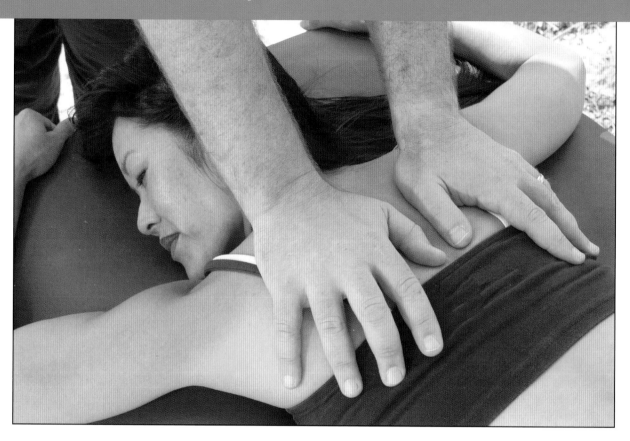

What the Technique Does

Reduces upper back and shoulder stiffness and discomfort.

Why It Works

This technique releases tension, which remains in the trapezius muscles after you apply Technique 5. Additionally, it helps reduce the tightness in the muscles lying on the surface of the scapula (your shoulder blade), and in the small muscles between the ribs.

How It Is Done

Place your hands on your partner's upper back with the heel of your hand (the thick meaty part at the base of your thumb) in the middle of the shoulder blades with your fingers pointed toward her lower back. Apply pressure evenly through the palm of your hand, and slightly less in the fingers, in a direction down into the table or floor and toward her buttocks. Let the pressure be a gentle pulse, following her breathing, applying pressure when she exhales and releasing when she inhales.

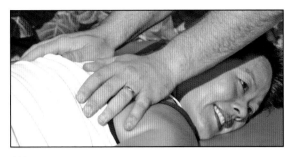

Hint

This technique is great for an upper respiratory infection or cold. The rib mobilization can greatly relieve the discomfort associated with constant coughing, although it should not be performed during active coughing.

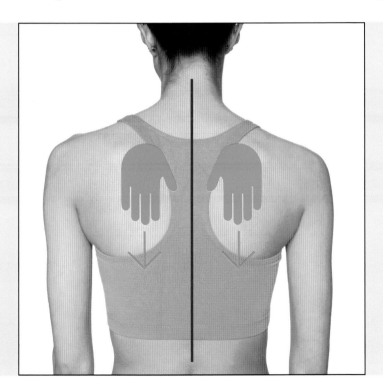

Basic Prone Thoracic Release

What the Technique Does:

Helps reduce thoracic and upper back discomfort.

Why It Works

There are several large muscle groups in this area. In the upper portion of the thoracic spine you will apply pressure to the lower reaches of the trapezius muscle, as well as the rhomboids. In the lower portions, you will be on top of the latissmus dorsi and serratus muscles. Additionally, this technique indirectly releases the intercostal muscles between the ribs. Relaxing them and indirectly mobilizing the thoracic vertebrae helps restore normal movement to this area of the spine and alleviate soft tissue tenderness as well.

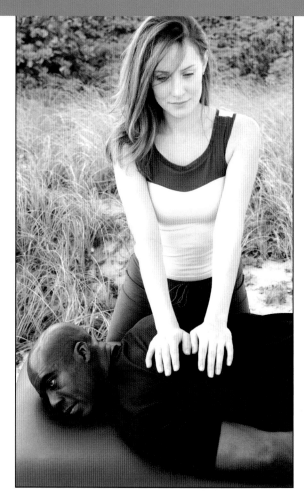

How It Is Done

With the heels of your hands just lateral to the spinous processes running down the center of the back and your fingers pointing outwards, apply slow gentle pressure down through the table and away from the spine. Your pulsations should again mirror your partner's breathing—applying pressure when she exhales, and slowly releasing as she inhales. Note that you are working on the side opposite from where you are located (if you are on your partner's left side, apply pressure to the right side of her spine and vice versa).

Hint:

Try placing your fingers in between your partner's ribs as you begin to apply pressure. This will help to relax these small muscles even more effectively. Also, try to feel her rib movement as she breathes. As you become more adept at palpation, you may notice some ribs moving more smoothly than others, and how all of the rib movement can normalize as you apply your techniques.

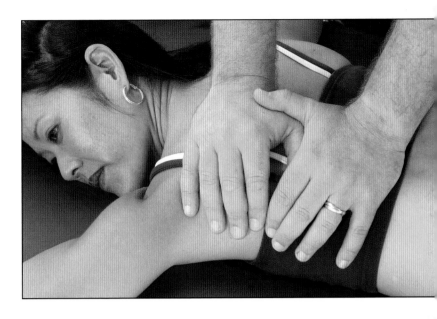

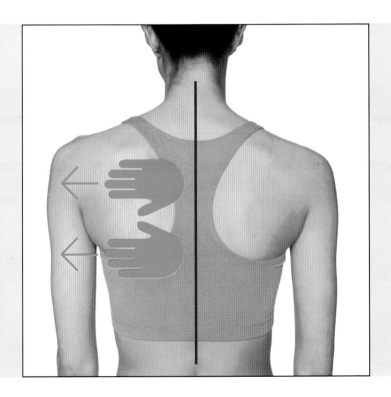

Following each application, work your way lower and lower down the thoratic spine.

Simple Thoracic Mobilization and Release

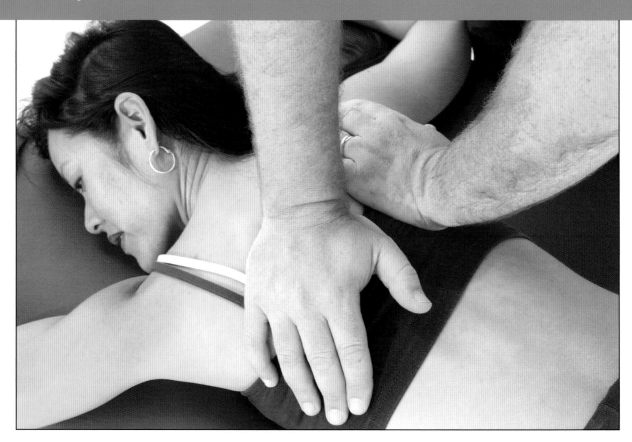

What the Technique Does

This maneuver helps to restore normal movement of the thoracic spine and ribs, decreasing midback pain.

Why It Works

Daily activities can sometimes cause dysfunction of these vertebrae and restrict movement, resulting in pain. This approach introduces both side-bending and rotation to the segments of the thoracic spine, helping restore normal movement.

How It Is Done

Standing next to your partner, place one hand on either side of her thoracic spine (as always, being careful not to apply pressure to the spinous processes), with one hand's fingers pointing toward the head, and the other pointing toward the tailbone. Apply even pressure, with the force going through into the table and into the direction of your fingers. Gradually apply pressure with exhalation and slowly release with inhalation. When this group of vertebrae relaxes, move your hands down a few vertebrae and repeat. When you have covered the vertebrae going in one direction, reverse the direction of your hands and repeat the procedure going the other way.

Hint

This is one of those techniques where you may occasionally feel or hear a "crack." This is not bad or dangerous, and conversely should not be the goal of your technique.

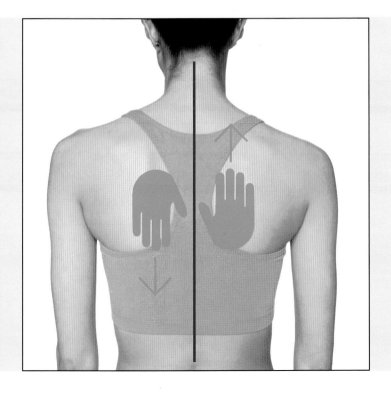

Basic Prone Lumbar Release

What the Technique Does

Reduces lumbar discomfort and stiffness.

Why It Works

There are several large muscle groups in this area of the spine, including the lower portion of the latiss-mus dorsi, the erector spinae, iliocostalis, and longissmus muscles. They support and move the

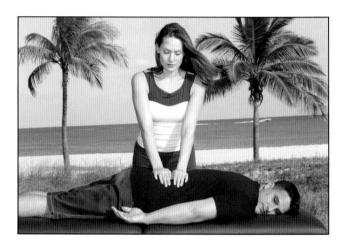

majority of the weight of your upper body; they are therefore worked hard on a daily basis and are susceptible to tension as well as minor strain during regular use. Additionally, a sedentary lifestyle can contribute to dysfunction of the vertebrae of the lumbar spine. This technique helps mobilize and restore normal function to these segments.

How It Is Done

This technique is remarkably similar to the Prone Thoracic Release (Technique 7) and is almost as easy; the primary difference between the techniques is that these muscles support a greater amount of body mass, and are therefore larger, so more pressure may be required to achieve the desired results. With your hands next to each other, apply pressure just alongside the spinous processes down and away from your partner's center, increasing pressure gradually as she exhales and slowly releasing when she inhales. You will feel these muscles become less tense and ropelike as you continue to apply your pressure. Depending upon the size of your hands and your partner's body, you may need to reorient your hand position several times to affect the entire lumbar spine.

Hint

Try combining this technique with the Simple Lumbar Mobilization (Technique 10) and the Sacral Flexion and Extension (Technique 11) to help reduce low back soreness, particularly after strenuous activity (such as shoveling snow).

Variation

These muscles get larger as you move down the spine, the same way a pyramid's base increases as you get closer to the bottom. This is a feat of natural engineering. Sometimes it helps to increase the pressure you apply to this area by stacking one hand on top of the other as you get closer to the bottom of the lumbar spine.

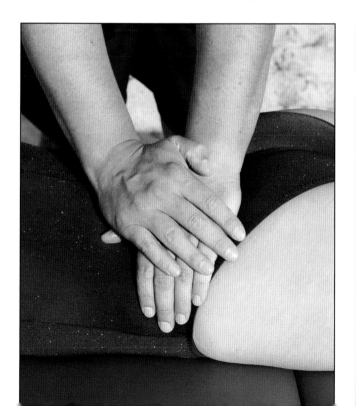

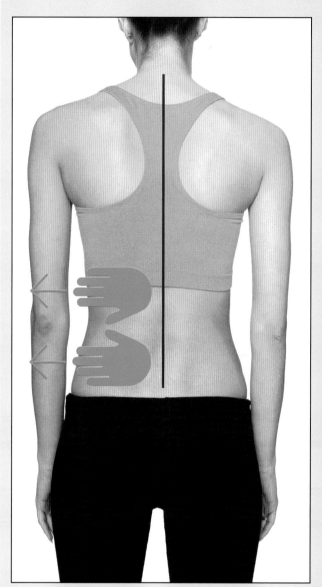

Simple Lumbar Mobilization and Release

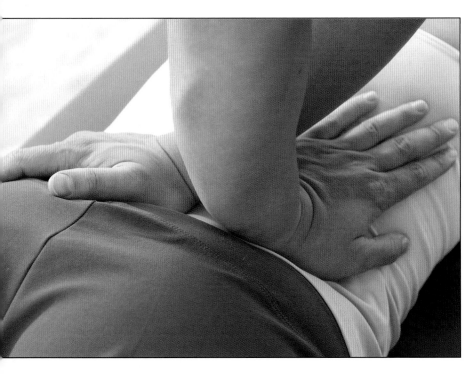

What the Technique Does

This helps restore normal movement to the vertebrae of the lumbar spine, and reduces muscle tension and soreness, alleviating low back discomfort.

Why It Works

Like the similar Simple Thoracic Mobilization (Technique 8), this technique introduces side-bending and rotation movement to the vertebrae of the lumbar spine. (Here's how to differentiate between the two: To bend, take your left hand and just bend to the left, sliding your hand down your thigh. To rotate, turn your shoulders to the back.)

How It Is Done:

Place your hands upon your partner's lumbar musculature alongside the spine, with one hand on either side and the fingers pointed in opposing directions. Apply pressure with her exhalation, down toward the floor and in the direction of your fingers. Release pressure with inhalation. Relocate your hands to move up and down the lumbar spine, and then switch the directions of your fingers to get side-bending in the opposite direction.

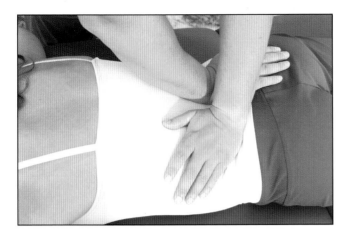

Hint:

These larger muscle groups may require more force as well as a longer application of the technique to achieve the desired result. You may notice that the muscles in this region of the back are more prone to resist side-bending movement. As you perform this maneuver, you will notice that the amount of pressure you need to apply gradually decreases.

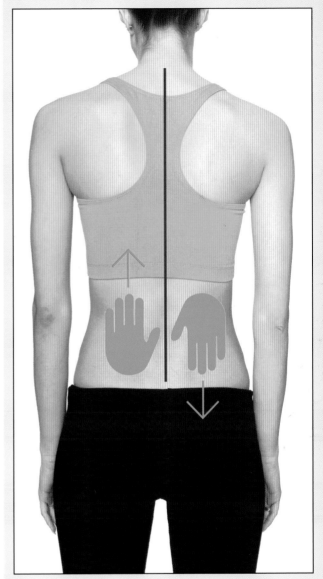

Sacral Flexion and Extension

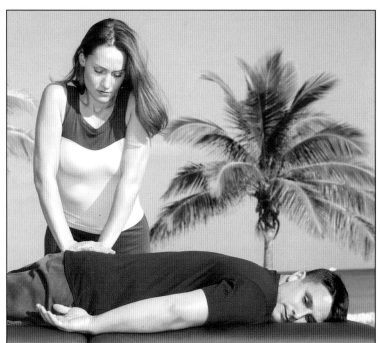 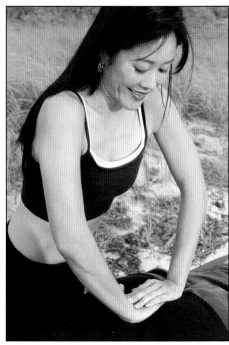

What the Technique Does

Reduces low back stiffness and soreness, and sacroiliac pain.

Why It Works

The sacrum is the "keystone" of your spine. It supports the total weight of your upper body and articulates the entire movement of walking. Extended periods of sitting put the sacrum in a flexed position and cause the associated muscles and ligaments to tighten up around it. The manual flexion and extension of the sacrum introduced by this technique help undo the effects of prolonged sitting, and restore normal movement to the sacrum and the sacroiliac joints (the juncture between the sacrum and the adjacent pelvic bones).

How It Is Done

This is one of the fundamental techniques of traditional Osteopathic treatment, and the only one in this book where you will place pressure directly upon the midline of the spine. Place the palm of your hand directly upon your partner's sacrum (you will be able to identify it as the broad, flattened bony area at the bottom of the spine), fingers pointing toward her head. The palm should rest comfortably on the sacrum, "cupping" it. Place your other hand on the first, with the fingers pointing in the opposite direction. Apply firm downward pressure into the sacrum, and shift your weight from your left leg to your right and back again. (If you are performing the technique on the floor and you are on your knees, you can still do this.) The shifting of weight will result in a "rocking" motion to the sacrum. Hold the sacrum at the extreme ends of this motion—leaning all the way toward the head, and back toward the feet. Repeat this movement until you feel your partner's sacrum move smoothly toward both extremes.

Hint

By stimulating a cluster of parasympathetic nerves that lie about the sacrum, this technique is very useful for reducing menstrual pain.

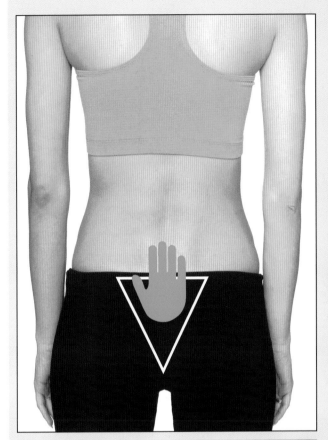

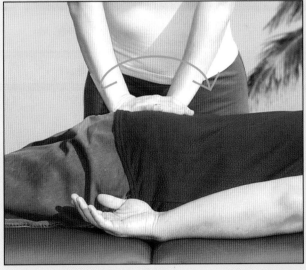

The Corner

What the Technique Does

Reduces low back and sacroiliac pain. Also reduces lumbar stiffness.

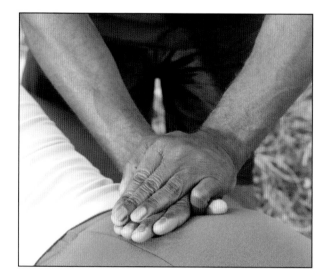

Why It Works

"The Corner" further relaxes the lumbar musculature and helps restore normal movement to the sacroiliac joint.

How It Is Done:

Initial hand position is key to getting results here. First, locate your partner's sacroiliac joint by following the sacrum to its edge where it meets the pelvic bone. You will feel a ridge between the two bones, which make up the sacroiliac joint. Place the palm of your hand just above the joint, on the thick lumbar muscles, with your fingertips lying across the sacrum and pointing at the opposite thigh. Place your other hand on top of the first. Apply pressure down and toward the opposite thigh. You should feel your palm "hook" over the edge of the pelvic bone. Follow your partner's breathing with the standard application of pressure.

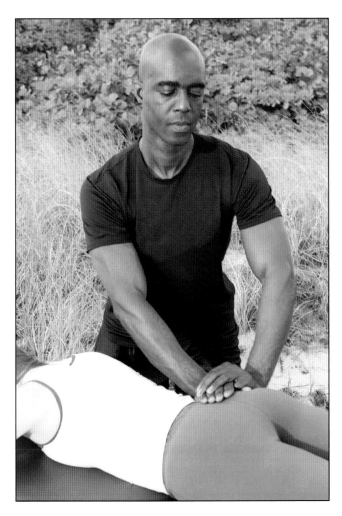

Hint:

The muscle relaxation you are trying to achieve here will not be as immediately apparent as in other maneuvers. Rely upon your partner's feedback to help you determine how long you should perform the technique. Also try combining this technique with the Sacral Flexion and Extension (Technique 11) for sacroiliac discomfort.

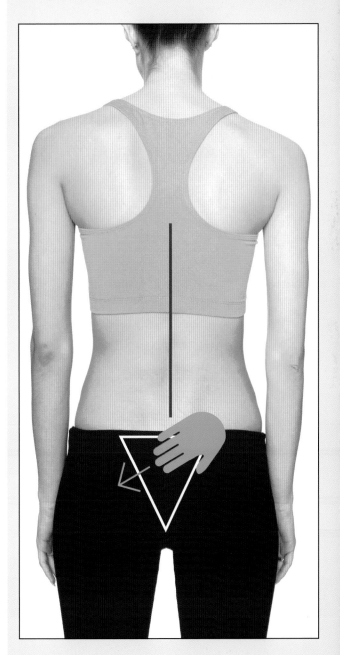

Basic Piriformis Release

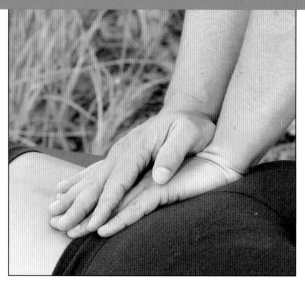

What the Technique Does

The piriformis release can be useful in reducing sciatic pain, as well as restoring normal movement to the sacrum.

Why It Works

The piriformis is a short, thick band of muscle that crosses the space between the sacrum and the hip. When this muscle is tense or goes into spasm, it can irritate the sciatic nerve that lies just underneath it, causing sciatic pain (the kind of pain that shoots down the back of the leg). Spasm in this muscle can also limit adequate movement of the sacrum, resulting in low back discomfort.

How It Is Done

Place your hand in the central part of the buttocks, with the heel of your hand just below the lower edge of the sacrum. Apply slow, even pressure directly into the thickest region of the buttocks with your force going toward the sacrum. This time, you need not vary your pressure with your partner's respiration. Instead, apply steady pressure to the tense region in the central area of the cheek until you feel the muscle relax.

Just a quick note on the importance of hand position in this and the preceding technique: In "The Corner" (Technique 12), your hand is **above** the sacrum, with your fingers pointing **down** towards the opposite thigh. When performing the Piriformis Release, the hand is **below** the sacrum, with the fingertips pointing **up** toward your partner's opposite armpit.

Hint:

This area commonly becomes tender and can develop "trigger points" (small tender areas which, when irritated, can cause pain in the area of the point as well as a second location "triggered" by the irritation). If this occurs, you may find it helpful to "desensitize" your partner. This can be accomplished by placing the broad part of the palm on this same region and applying gentle, even pressure, slowly increasing, sometimes over minutes, until your partner can tolerate the deep pressure associated with the actual technique.

Try combining this approach with Sacral Flexion and Extension (Technique 11) and the Lumbar-Sacral Circle (Technique 14) to help reduce sciatic discomfort.

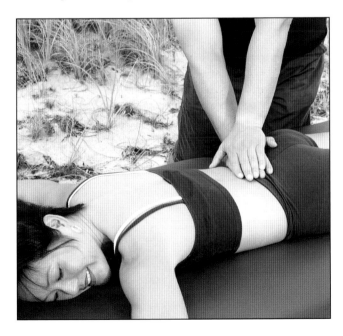

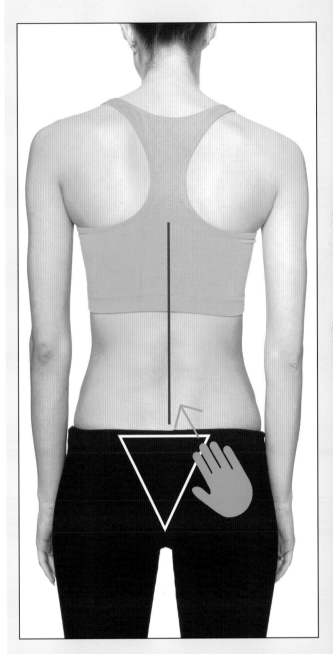

The Lumbar-Sacral Circle

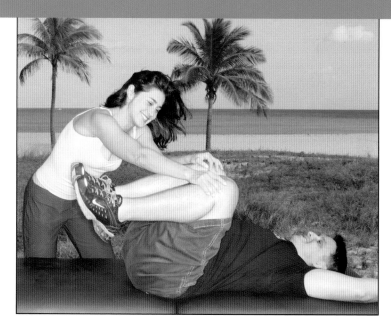

What the Technique Does

Reduces low back stiffness and soreness. It can be helpful in restoring normal function to the sacrum, especially when there is sacroiliac joint dysfunction and pain.

Why It Works

This is actually a mobilization technique, meaning that its benefit is achieved through movement of a joint or joints. In this case, the sacroiliac joints, as well as those of the lumbar spine, are all gently moved through a broad range of motion. Performing this maneuver on a firm surface will gently move the sacrum through flexion, extension, and left and right side-bending.

How It Is Done

This is a serious "bang for your buck" technique, as minimal experience on your part can still yield tremendous benefit for your partner. With your partner flat on his back, raise his knees until his thighs are perpendicular to the ground. Slowly move the knees around in a small circular pattern, a couple of times in each direction. After a few rotations, enlarge the circumference of your circles until his knees are approaching the plane of his chest. If his head represents the 12 o'clock position, pause to hold his knees in both the 10 and 2 o'clock positions, applying gentle pressure when you get to the largest circles.

Hint:

Combine this movement with Sacral Flexion and Extension (Technique 11) to further decrease menstrual pain. This movement also replicates the movements of some traditional Osteopathic lymphatic drainage techniques, so try combining it with the Prone Trapezius/Rib Release (Technique 6) to reduce the symptoms of an upper respiratory infection or bronchitis.

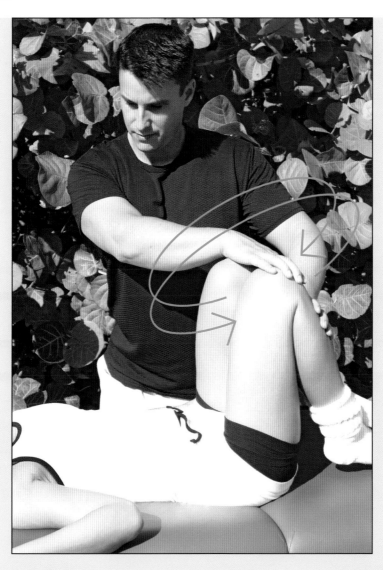

Elbow Circle Thoracic Mobilization

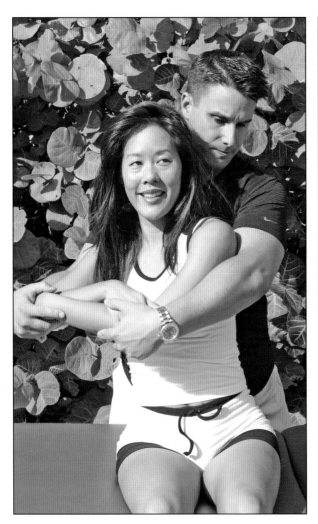 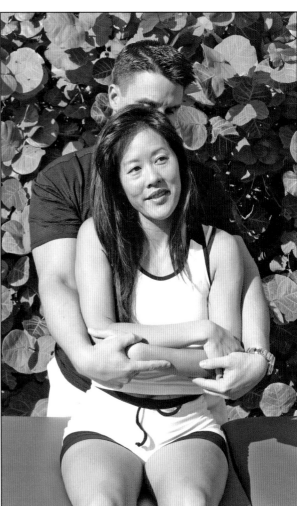

What the Technique Does:

Use this technique to reduce thoracic and shoulder stiffness. It also helps gently mobilize the thoracic vertebrae.

Why It Works

At first glance, this technique appears to be somewhat out of order, but it is in fact remarkably similar in concept and execution to the Lumbar-Sacral Circle (Technique 14). Its circular motion gently mobilizes the upper thoracic spine through flexion, extension, and side-bending movements. Additionally, it moves the shoulders through a broad range of motion.

How It Is Done

While standing behind your seated partner, ask her to clasp her hands on her elbows. Reaching around her torso, grab her elbows, and with her back against your chest, begin to move the elbows in a circular pattern, with the center of her chest as the axis. Gradually increase the size of the circles until her forearms nearly touch her forehead. As in the previous technique, be sure to introduce the movement in both directions.

Variation

If your partner is significantly larger than you, seat her with her back against a wall. While standing in front of her, perform the same range of movement.

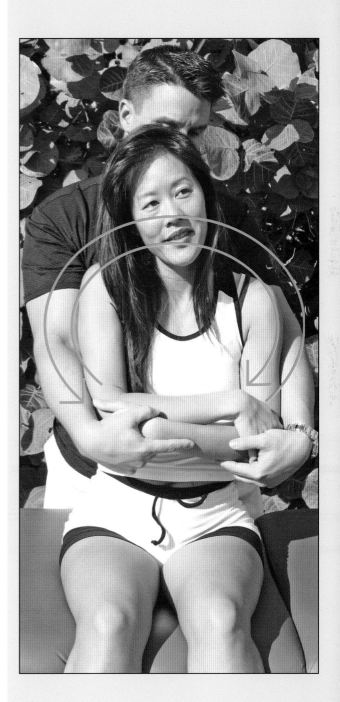

Shoulder Circle Scapular Mobilization

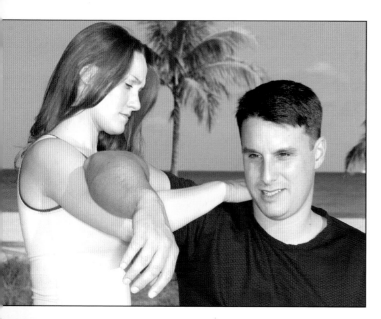

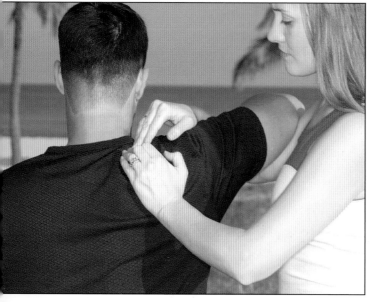

What the Technique Does

This maneuver reduces shoulder stiffness and pain, as well as reducing discomfort in the thoracic spine.

Why It Works

There are several thick, short muscles beneath the scapula (the flat, triangular bone of your shoulder blade.) The connective tissue associated with these muscles is intermingled with that of the upper thoracic spine and ribs. When muscle tension affects one of these regions, the other areas are affected as well. This approach helps by moving the scapula through a broad range of motion, and relaxing the muscles attached to it, including the supraspinatus and infraspinatus.

How It Is Done

I saved this one for last, as the hand position is a little trickier than in previous techniques. Stand at the side of your seated partner, facing him, or sit next to him so that your shoulders and his are approximately the same height. Place your arm closest to your partner underneath his armpit so that your hand rests comfortably on the back of his shoulder. Take your free hand and line up your fingers so that they are touching the fingers on your other hand right on top of the "belly" of the trapezius (essentially the same point you located for the Seated Trapezius Release, Technique 5). Your palm should rest on the shoulder blade itself.

Once you have the hand position straight, the actual technique is simple: Using the forearm you have looped under your partner's armpit, move his arm in small circles forward and backward while pressing down on the belly of the trapezius. The palms should be applying pressure through your partner, toward his chest.

Hint

As I related earlier, the hand position in this technique can appear complicated until you have done it a few times. Try practicing the "set up" on each other to become more comfortable with it before you actually apply the technique.

Variation

Some individuals with a rotator cuff injury, or who have had shoulder surgery, may not be able to tolerate having their arm extended outward all the way. If this is the case, stand slightly closer to your partner so that his upper arm is at a lesser angle. You can then do the rest of the technique the same way.

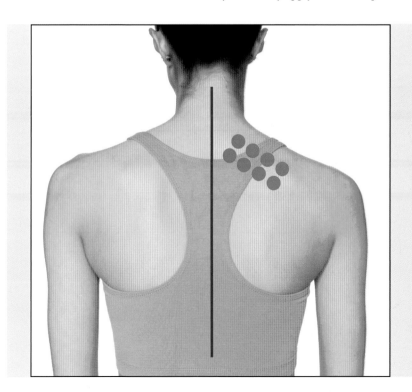

Habits and Habitus

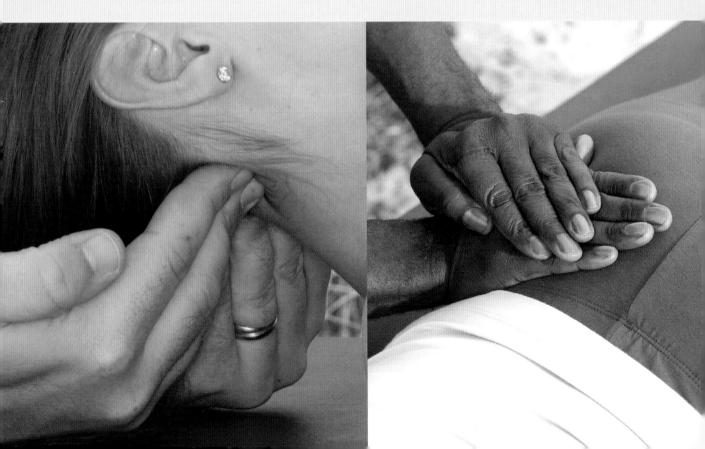

What the heck does "habitus" mean?

So many factors contribute to painful conditions, I could spend an eternity trying to outline them all. However, you have direct and immediate control over several of them. You have spent the past several sections learning about physical and psychological factors, as well as simple hands-on approaches with which you can help alleviate discomfort. Now let's take a look at some of the home and workplace variables that you can manipulate in order to achieve a higher quality of pain-free life.

It has probably become clear to you that your habits have a tremendous effect on the frequency and severity of the pain you will experience. These habits represent the first link in the chain of what I refer to as the four H's:

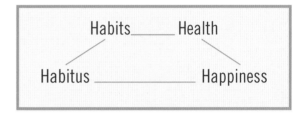

Previously, we defined the Triad of Pain. In this section we will examine what I refer to as the Trapezoid of Well-Being (yes, I actually did write that).

The Triad of Pain focused on the elements that cause and augment pain; the four H's focus on the elements that contribute to making you feel better.

While you are probably familiar with habits, health, and happiness, you probably are not familiar with the word "habitus." It refers to your physical body, where you live. It is affected both by genetic factors (including inherited diseases and traits such as a tendency towards high cholesterol) over which you have no control, and overall health as dictated by diet, exercise, sleep, stress levels—largely mediated by personal habits. Your habits, health, and habitus influence your overall happiness, so you can see how they are all tied together.

We will talk about habits in the home and workplace a little bit later. Here I would like to focus on what I perceive as the most important habit you can create: a regular fitness routine.

I know that it can be difficult to even imagine exercise when you are in pain. When I was dealing with the back pain I experienced after my car accident, the last thing I wanted to think about was exercising. However, it is easy to identify the clear benefits of exercise on both the actual level of pain and the way you experience it. Among them are:

- Improved range of motion
- Increased muscle strength
- Increased cardiovascular endurance
- Stress reduction
- Better oxygenation of tissue
- Endorphin release

When dealing with pain that likely has a mechanical origin, it is easy to see why exercise would be so important. What is less clear is how one gets motivated enough to get off one's can and actually start to work out.

It is important to understand, first and foremost, that exercise does not necessarily mean hardcore weightlifting and long-distance running. A good stretching routine and a walk can have incredible, positive benefit. The question is how to introduce a routine without incurring major setbacks.

Again, this is an area where working with your partner will likely yield greater benefits than trying to throw yourself at this endeavor on your own. Presumably, by this point you, the pain sufferer, know what's wrong, and have a correct diagnosis. You understand which activities make the pain better or worse. Your partner is probably developing an idea of what your limits are. With this in mind, you should both sit down and discuss your options. Take out a sheet of paper, and address some of these concerns:

1. When will you exercise? Choose a schedule you can both commit to and live with on a regular basis. This is often the primary factor in whether exercise becomes a regular part of your life. If

you can really push yourself to adhere to the schedule for at least the first few weeks, exercise will likely become a habit rather than something you have to push yourself to start. One of the nice things about regular exercise is that its effects on your discomfort are often very immediate and profound, providing additional motivation for you to continue.

2. Discuss your fitness goals. Do you have a weak area that needs to be strengthened? Are you trying to lose weight? Are you simply trying to become "more fit"? Is it likely that increasing your core strength (those muscles around your spine, torso, and abdominals) will decrease your back pain?

3. What sort of exercise will you do? Do you have any fitness equipment in your home? Will you go to a fitness club?

4. How are you going to motivate each other? How will you differentiate between the belief that you "hurt too much" to exercise today, and the reality that you probably can still work out? How can your partner also learn to tell the difference? This too will be a learning process which may take some time to establish.

There are other questions to ask, but these will vary depending upon your particular situation.

Like any other activities that you may introduce while trying to reduce your pain level, exercise needs to be introduced in a methodical, "as-tolerated" fashion. Everyone has different tolerances, and depending upon your exercise needs and goals, the way your exercise program evolves will initially depend upon both of you, but hopefully your ability to continue to reap the benefits of your program will gradually depend less and less upon your partner.

Weight

Heaven knows, popular media has rammed the issue of maintaining proper weight down the throats of Americans for years. In spite of this fact, obesity continues to be an increasing nationwide health problem. In response to this epidemic, thousands of products have been created promising to help reduce weight. I have had to deal with my own food and weight issues.

With regard to back pain, this item very much needs to be dealt with. The spine, being essentially a mechanical device, is subject to stress through use. Increasing this stress by adding weight can compromise its functioning in broad, far-reaching ways. In my practice, I have observed that a large proportion of back pain can be reduced simply by achieving an appropriate weight for your body type. Achieving optimal weight can improve pain from arthritis and disc disease. Additionally, the emotional benefits from improved body image will enhance feeling of well-being. How you get there is based upon your personal situation, but this issue clearly deserves your attention.

Clothes Make the Man and Woman

It's remarkable that something as fundamental as clothing can have such a profound affect on the way we all feel. We all get dressed in the morning, but how many of us actually give consideration to the physiologic effects of our clothes? Here are a few ways to make sure that the clothing you wear does not adversely impact the way you feel.

Some of these items are gender specific, so feel free to bounce around a little.

Pants

Most men like to feel they can wear the same size pants they wore in college, or when they got married, but often times this isn't the case. As a man's waist gets larger, his pants get lower and lower on his hips until his belt sits right on his sacroiliac joint, impeding its movement in profound ways. A study of 100 randomly selected men in my practice demonstrated that over 50 percent of them regularly wear pants that are the wrong size (almost always too small).

Pants size should be measured annually (more often if there has been considerable weight loss or gain), and the size you purchase should be correct and honest. If you are truly unhappy with your waist size, there are better ways of addressing it than lying to yourself and getting a size smaller than appropriate. In addition to placing undue pressure on the sacroiliac joint, the wrong pants size can alter breathing mechanics and affect the flexion and extension of the lumbar spine.

Jackets

Jackets should be fitted properly. A tight jacket will pull across the shoulders and impede correct thoracic movement. Measure yourself annually, and purchase the correct size. If you are not sure whether something fits correctly, make sure it buttons well; any rear vents or splits in the jacket should not be pulled apart, and the buttons should not appear tugged.

Pull both arms across to the opposite shoulders. The jacket should not tug across the back. Avoid heavier coats, particularly those that are asymmetrical in their construction. And last, don't pack your pockets with all manner of paraphernalia that could weigh you down and place unnecessary stress on your neck and shoulders.

Bras

In 2002, we examined 150 women patients. (They were not randomly selected; you would be surprised by how many did not want to be measured.) We asked a female medical student, who had learned the correct techniques for bra sizing from "fitting experts" at a major department store and a lingerie specialty store, to measure this sample of our patients. Over 50 percent were wearing the wrong size bra, and of those women, over 70 percent had a somatic dysfunction of their thoracic spine at or near the level where their bra crossed over their back.

However, once I determined that most women had a problem with the way they were fitted for their bras, I was at a loss to provide any useful advice beyond recommending the correct size. I was clearly not in a position to speak from personal experience. I went to lingerie stores to see if sales associates could provide any useful information. While most of them agreed on the correct way to measure bra size, few could agree on a style that was most comfortable and offered the most support. Sometimes, the discussion started heated debate between saleswomen. There seemed to be consensus that styles that used broader expanses of fabric in their cups and wider straps to distribute the weight of the breasts tended to be more comfortable, but were also considered uglier by the women who recommended them. The bottom line is, correct size and good support add up to fewer back problems.

Underpants

Always wear clean underpants. This just seems like a good idea. I have nothing constructive to add here, but the word "underpants" is just so gosh darn funny (as opposed to the word "underwear," which isn't funny at all—don't ask me why).

Shoes

Shoes could actually account for their own book, so let's stick with some basic recommendations:

Look at the bottoms of a pair of shoes you have had for a long time. The soles will show greater wear in the areas that sustain the greatest abuse. There should be even wear over the heel and midsole, but there rarely is. If you notice that the outer or inner edges of your shoes are disproportionately more worn than the other surfaces, your feet may be either pronated or supinated (leaning in or out irregularly). If this is the case, the arch of the foot cannot do its job properly—that is, absorb shocks before they can go up your leg and into your spine. This situation can generally be rectified with the use of orthotic inserts (great in sneakers, walking shoes, and boots—not so good in heels!), which

are easily obtained from a qualified podiatrist. Orthotics can cost a few hundred dollars, but are usually a one-time investment (sometimes covered by medical insurance) and will save you a world of pain later on.

Athletic shoes are designed not only to protect your feet but also to absorb the shock associated with exercise that would impact your spine. The correct size is supremely important. Beyond that, there are a few things to consider. Make sure you have chosen the appropriate shoe for the type of exercise you routinely do. Shoe designers put a lot of thought into how different rubber compounds and materials cope with the stresses of various sports. A walking shoe will have distinctly different dynamic properties from a basketball shoe. Also, don't wear shoes for too long. The various compounds in their soles eventually become so compressed from overuse that they lose their ability to absorb impact. Depending upon how much activity you do, six to nine months is probably the longest you should use a pair of athletic shoes (somewhat less if you also use them as "leisure" shoes for daily wear).

High Heels

Heels get a bad rap. People have been told that heels are bad and therefore avoid them altogether. Good news, they aren't so bad after all. Actually, moderately high heels (1 to $1^1/_2$ inches) can actually be beneficial to your back by helping to maintain the correct lumbar lordotic curve (the curve that makes your butt stick out) **provided that** they have a broad base. Stiletto heels, while attractive, create an unstable base from which to propel yourself while walking, or to balance yourself. Mules usually have a good, wide heel with plenty of surface area. I wear cowboy boots almost all the time, and the one-inch heel has always been comfortable and easy on my back.

Accessories

Belts

Follow the same basic rules you would with pants: not too tight, not sitting on the sacrum.

Bags

The Number One accessory enemy of the spine is the bag you carry. Handbags, book bags, satchels, or purses are invariably overloaded, mostly with items you don't even remember are in there. Therefore, the first recommendation is to pare down the contents to what you actually need with you. After you have done this, see if what you have is still disproportionately heavy. School-age children are particularly susceptible to this diabolical method of spinal torture. Try picking up your kid's book bag. You may be amazed at how much she is schlepping around on a daily basis!

Next, look at the ergonomics of the bag itself. A handgrip handle is probably the worst if the load is moderately heavy. A same-shoulder strap is slightly less damaging. A strap across the shoulder is the safest bet for distributing the weight in a non-destructive fashion.

Collars and Ties

The tie can be grouped with collared shirts inasmuch as the fit around the cervical spine can make the difference between painless and painful. As with pants, some people don't want to acknowledge the changes their bodies undergo over time, and frequently wear collars and ties that are too tight and restrict cervical movement. A poorly fitting collar can cause neck pain and severe headaches, as well as having consequences for the remainder of the spine.

The bottom line is, clothing makes a difference. It's easy to gravitate toward the items we think are fashionable or cost effective. Next time you go shopping, think about the clothes you buy and their effects on your spine. You can be a thrifty fashion plate and still stand up straight.

A Brief Note About Picking Up Children

Carrying children is one of the most fundamental ways parents have to comfort, console, and bond with their kids. If you have children, one of the most frustrating aspects of living with back pain is its dramatic change in your ability to interact with them. If they are newborns or infants, your natural instinct is to hold them, and the long-term benefits derived from "attachment parenting" (where the child is carried as often as possible, kept close to the primary caregivers) are widely known. If they are toddlers or older, you already know that even when you are exhausted, your child wants to be picked up—it is one of the ways children cope with their own discomfort. Children have expectations about the people around

them, and not meeting those expectations can affect parent-child relationships in powerful, damaging ways. I don't suggest that if you have back pain you will necessarily have a bad relationship with your children. What I am saying is that you have tools and methods to prevent this from becoming an issue.

There are some basic guidelines to carrying your child that will save you lots of grief:

1. Portable bassinets are perfectly fine for providing your child a place to rest or sleep when you go out. They are **horrible** for carrying your child from place to place. No matter how manufacturers try to offset the handle and provide an ergonomic solution to the "baby-bucket," they offset the weight too far away from the carrier's center of gravity. This causes the lumbar spine to shift, exacerbates low back discomfort, and in time causes new problems.

2. Use your hips. Both women and men can carry a child on their side, using their hips for support. Having the child's legs straddle the hip just above the pelvic bone will provide a stable base close to

the carrier's center of gravity, and prevent all sorts of mayhem.

3. A sling, front carrier, or baby backpack is an outstanding method to transport a child without unnecessarily endangering your spine. Front carriers tend to be best for newborn and infant children. Slings have the benefit of maintaining their usefulness from infancy all the way through toddlerhood (my daughter now carries her doll around in a sling). This device allows the child to remain at close to eye level with the adult, and studies suggest that this closeness may enhance early childhood social development.

4. Switch sides. It is easy to get into the habit of holding your child on one side or the other. Switch and give each side a little break.

5. You probably already know that taking a baby out generally requires lots and lots of paraphernalia: diaper bags, bottles, strollers, toys, mats, the whole kit and kaboodle. This may seem like common sense, but try to consolidate what you really need

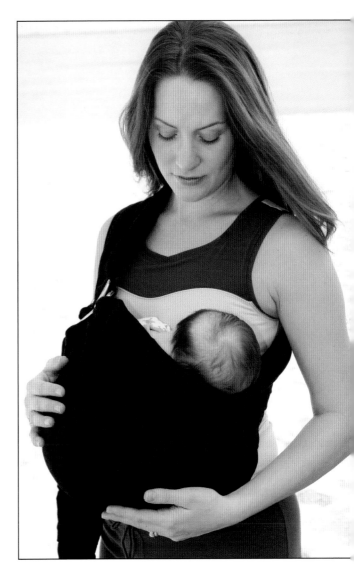

into a small, truly portable container. My wife put a spare diaper and a change of clothing into the bottom of the sling. Her sling doubled as a changing mat, and she didn't need to haul along a stroller.

6. If your painful condition precludes your carrying your child, set her on your lap as often as possible to make up for the difference. The closeness will make you feel better, and she will not feel let down by your inability to carry her. In this case, a stroller is a sensible alternative, as you can push the baby without having to support its weight, and all the accessories can be tucked underneath (my wife suggests alternating having the baby face you with facing the rest of the world). In this case, try to get down to eye level with your child by sitting or squatting next to the stroller as often as possible to help re-establish the connection between the two of you.

7. When you do pick up your children, particularly as they progress from infants into toddlerhood, remember to use good lifting technique. Bend at your knees, hug your child close to your center of gravity, and lift using your legs. Limit the time that you are actually supporting her weight to a period shorter than it would take to begin to feel discomfort. Then you either put her down or sit with her on your lap to extend the close time.

8. Once you have begun to address the underlying causes of your pain, consider picking up your kids as part of your treatment plan. Pick them up once or twice a day, and gradually increase the amount of time you spend to raise your tolerance. You may find that your overall strength will increase, and you will begin to find this holding time is part of your recovery rather than an activity to be avoided. This will provide the multifaceted benefit of affecting the physiologic, the learned neurological response, and the psychological amplifier all at once.

Hi Ho, Hi Ho: Work

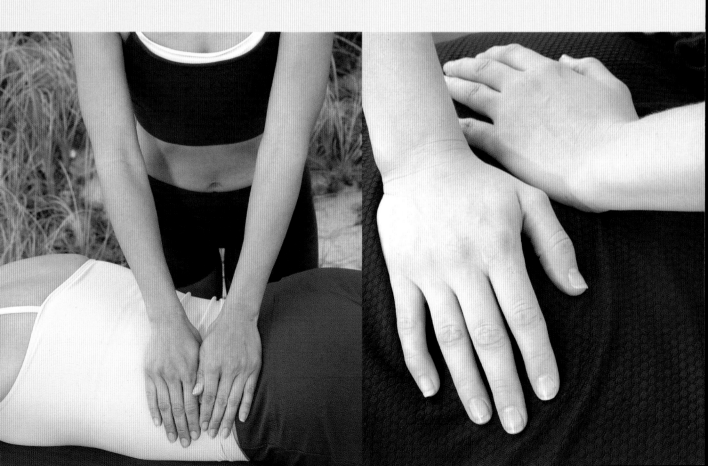

People spend a lot of time at their desks, either at work or at home. As you already know, sitting on your butt for hours a day is horrible for your spine. We can prove this by examining jobs that require much sitting; statistically, secretaries and typists are the most likely professions to experience back pain, after truckers. Unfortunately, many of us have little choice in the matter—either because of work, or home administrative responsibilities, or maybe even helping our kids with their homework. Whatever your reason is, I can state with certainty that most of you sit too much. Therefore, let's optimize sit-down time to minimize the damage.

From time to time, patients have asked me to do an ergonomic assessment of their work environments. While I have found that almost *all* of these workplaces are seriously compromised, a few simple changes would improve them significantly.

Take a look at your desk. Where is everything? Did you put conscious thought into the placement of the objects that cover it? Or, more likely, did they all wind up in random places, or in locations that were either aesthetically pleasing or completely unplanned? How about your chair? Did you measure your chair and determine if it was constructed to give you optimum height and support? Or was it on sale at your local office supply store (the most common response)? Maybe it matched your other furniture. You probably spend enough time at your desk to warrant an examination of these issues and more. If you share your workspace with others, or with a spouse at home, you can do many things which don't necessarily cost a lot of money or require a tremendous amount of effort, but which greatly improve your situation.

The Chair

Seated posture is perhaps the most important factor in reducing back pain in the office. Knowing this, there are obvious reasons to put some thought into this purchase. If you are in a workplace with a chair provided to you, your employer should be willing to purchase (or reimburse you for) ergonomically appropriate seating. If they are not, it would still be beneficial in the long run to purchase on your own. Here are some helpful guidelines in selecting a chair:

1. Try to get an adjustable-height chair, so you can obtain optimal height no matter what work you are doing. Writing may require a different position than working at your computer. If you share a desk with someone else, this will enable both of you to identify a correct work posture. Optimal height is essentially determined by the position of your feet on the ground—your feet should rest flat on the floor, with your shins vertical and your thighs horizontal.

2. Choose a chair with a back support. Some manufactures have marketed stools that are supposed to help promote healthy posture. They may be useful when you are at your best and actively thinking about your posture. In truth, you don't think about it most of the time, and if you are a little fatigued, your posture probably tends toward the lousy. A backrest will at least offer some support and a guideline for better posture. If the backrest is ergonomically designed and offers lumbar support, all the better.

3. Get a rolling chair. This provides access to all parts of the desk and will discourage you from stretching across the desk for something out of reach. It's better to condition yourself to shift the chair a few inches in each direction in order to get to objects on your desktop.

4. Make sure the chair can get close enough to the desk to optimize your work position. Many chairs have high armrests that keep you from putting them close to the desk. In this case, you wind up sliding your butt to the front edge of the chair, thereby negating any benefit the backrest might have offered.

The Computer

The computer has simplified many complicated office tasks. Its ubiquitous position in our homes and workplaces has also introduced a whole host of musculoskeletal dysfunctions. At work we tend to be bound to our computers for any number of work-related activities, and when we go home, the Internet has replaced the television as a source of evening entertainment for many people. While this amount of computer time is arguably unhealthy for other reasons, it needn't be with regards to your spinal well-being. There are three things to consider.

1. The monitor: It should be as close to eye level as possible, putting your cervical spine in a neutral position and far enough away from your face to avoid straining your eyes. Many people, however, place their monitors on their desks without any risers underneath, putting their necks in a flexed position for hours at a time. Additionally, your monitor should be placed directly above the keyboard. I am amazed at how many offices I've seen where the monitor was pushed off to the side and the person sat at their desk with her head cocked in one direction or another (often with a telephone wedged between her ear and her shoulder). Simply correcting this one positional problem can greatly reduce the incidence of neck pain and headaches, as well as the visual fatigue associated with extended computer use. Also, if you stare at your computer monitor for long periods of time, occasionally look around the room in order to move your head into different positions and allow your eyes to focus on objects at different distances to save your eyesight.

2. The mouse: The computer's graphical user interface relies upon the use of the mouse. While it greatly simplifies computer use, it is also a danger to many who use it daily. It is very important to position your mouse in a way that does not force you to reach across your desk to use it. Conversely, placing your mouse too close will fatigue your shoulder unnecessarily. Try to position your mouse so that your forearm, your wrist, and the top of your hand are parallel with the desktop. And if possible, try to switch hands

periodically. Additionally, I have found that an alternative to the mouse is a trackball with a very large ball, or better yet a pen-based touch-pad, which accurately reproduces the writing movements you have been utilizing for most of your life. If you have been using a mouse for a long time these options may take some getting used to, but they can often prove beneficial in the long-term goal of reducing your musculoskeletal discomfort.

3. The keyboard: If you do a fair amount of typing, the position of your keyboard can have a greater effect on the well-being of your neck, shoulders, and wrists than any other modification you can make. Again, try to place the keyboard at a level which allows your hands, wrists, and forearms to remain parallel to the desktop.

There are numerous alternative-configuration keyboards available that you can use to optimally position your hands to decrease fatigue and prevent overuse ailments such as carpal tunnel syndrome. I have found that individuals need to investigate which ones are best for their own particular work habits and typing styles. My wife swears by her keyboard, which was designed for touch typists by splitting the left and right hand letters into separate sections. I **hate** it—I am a hunt-and-peck typist so it simply doesn't work for me. The experience of my patients supports this person-by-person variation. I encourage people to find a computer store with a liberal return policy, and "test drive" some of the keyboard alternatives.

You Are Sitting Too Much

As I mentioned previously, we as a culture tend to sit too much. No matter how much you optimize the accoutrements of your workspace, this one fact can completely undermine your efforts to feel well. Whether you are driving for a long distance, taking a long airplane flight, or sitting at your desk at home or work, the flexion of your spine in that sitting position needs to be reversed periodically to prevent both short- and long-term problems. Whenever you are going to sit for a long period of time, schedule yourself times to stand up and move, even if only for a few seconds. If you need to be reminded, set an alarm on your computer or clock to go off every half hour or so.

Your Telephone

If I could provide you with the one piece of work-place-related ergonomic advice that you must heed, it would be to get a telephone headset. At the very least, completely refrain from jamming your phone handset in between your ear and your shoulder. This is especially true if you use a cellular phone, because its relative thinness forces you to cock your head even farther toward one direction or another. There is almost nothing short of falling down a flight of stairs at your workplace that will disrupt the normal function of your cervical spine faster than holding your phone this way. Please find an alternative— **today**. Most cellular phones can be adapted with a hands-free headset for less than ten dollars. It may be somewhat more expensive to add a headset to your workplace phone, but it is well worth the investment.

Your Back's Top Ten

The following is my Double Secret Top Ten list of things you can do to reduce the effects of back pain in your life. If you do nothing else in this book, do these!

1. Buy a cordless headset for your telephone or cell phone. Not cradling the handset between your shoulder and ear will go farther than anything else you can do in your daily life to reduce neck discomfort.

2. If you carry a briefcase, purse, or book bag, go through the contents and see what you can do to lighten its weight. Do you need all of the items, or are you just carrying them due to habit? Try to regularly alternate the side on which you carry the bag.

3. If you sit for longer than an hour at a time, stand up and stretch out your legs and lower back. Remember, you weren't designed to sit nearly as much as you do.

4. Make sure your computer monitor, keyboard, and mouse are in the proper location. If you are sitting and staring at a computer monitor for much of the day, be sure to move your head into different positions periodically to avoid getting "stuck."

5. Try to maintain a body weight within 10 percent of your optimal body mass index (these figures are available in countless books and online).

6. Use proper lifting technique (lift with your legs—not with your back) when picking up heavy objects, your children, or any other items you may need to carry. While you are carrying them, keep the bulk of their mass close to your center of gravity (for example, place your children on your hip). Again, make an effort to alternate sides.

7. Get cardiovascular exercise at least four times a week. Try to vary the activity regularly. "Impact" activity done in moderation, such as jogging, can help prevent osteoporosis as well. Also, remember to stay adequately hydrated before, during, and after you exercise.

8. Get regular sleep. Quantity is not nearly as important as quality and regularity. Certainly don't go around sleep deprived; however, a good several hours of deep sleep is a lot more beneficial than a whole night of restless, shallow sleep.

9. Break up household tasks such as dusting and vacuuming into smaller, more manageable blocks. Maybe do one or two rooms a day rather than the whole house once per week.

10. Set aside a portion of every day to relax and unwind. Use this time to take a few deep breaths and recharge. Reflect upon your day and find a way to achieve your most calm state, even if for only a few moments. Again, quality over quantity. Use this time to acknowledge when you have not experienced pain today, or perhaps when it was not as severe as at other times.

Okay, Now What?

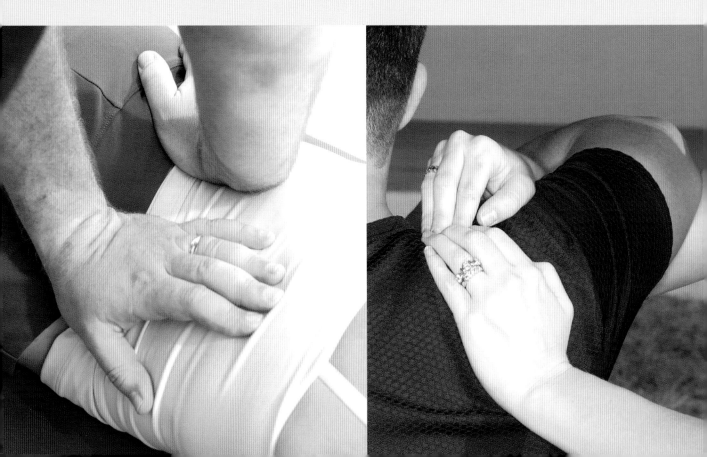

Now that you have some of the strategies, what are you going to do with them? At the beginning of this book, I said that I had looked at self-help books in depth (and remember that **this is not a self-help book**), and I noticed one glaring problem with many of them. Almost all ask you to significantly alter the way you normally do things—things which you may have been doing all of your life. For example, you may have always had a completely uncontrolled diet, and here's a book that tells you to eat nothing but tuna and sweet potatoes. How long will most people realistically stick with something like this? A radical action plan requires gradual implementation in order for you to stick with it. Considering all of the things we have discussed, how are you going to use them? It would be unrealistic of me to ask, or you to believe, that you will wake up tomorrow and do everything I

have recommended, and truthfully, that approach could do you more harm than good.

Remember that to one degree or another, almost everything we have discussed here involves learned behaviors and habits which have taken a long time to establish, and while some of them have caused you discomfort over time, your body has probably developed subconscious mechanisms to compensate for them. Trying to undo all of them at once would likely throw your compensatory mechanisms into disarray.

As usual, I will tell you right off the bat that the way you choose to implement some of the changes, strategies, and hands-on techniques I have outlined is an important and individual choice, to be based upon the specifics of your own circumstances. Here I will provide you a suggested framework that you can fine-tune and modify to suit your needs.

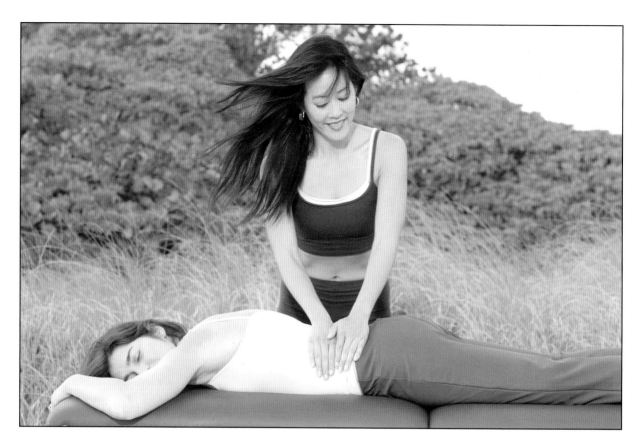

Before implementing any of the concepts in this book, work with your partner to complete a subjective pain assessment. Consider each of the regions in your body, and rate the level of pain you experience on a scale from 0 to 10. A sample assessment is provided on the right. No matter how much pain you are experiencing, do not be tempted to report 10 for any region unless it is really a 10—the most pain you can experience. Try to do the assessment three or four days in a row to get a rough average of what your condition actually looks like. One bad day could adversely affect your ability to accurately gauge your progress. In a few weeks you and your partner can look back at your initial assessment. Then you can see where you are going and what, if any, modifications to make to your program. Additionally, try to keep a diary of what you actually do during your implementation phase. It is easy to trick yourself into believing you are doing more than you actually are, so repeat the subjective pain assessment every few weeks.

Back Together: Hands-On Healing for Couples
Subjective Pain Assessment

Note: You may feel free to add or delete body regions as they apply to your personal pain profile.

Body Region	Week 1	Week 2	Week 3	Week 4	Week 5
Base of Skull					
Right Neck					
Left Neck					
Right Shoulder					
Left Shoulder					
Right Thoracic					
Left Thoracic					
Right Lumbar					
Left Lumbar					
Right Sacrum					
Left Sacrum					
Right Sciatic					
Left Sciatic					

A Sample Implementation Plan

Week 1

In any schedule you design, you and your partner should begin with a period of discussion. I recommend that you both read this book, or at least go through the techniques you are interested in using together. Discuss your needs and goals so that you can agree upon an effective implementation strategy.

Review the hands-on portion of this book, and introduce the first two techniques (p. 94 and p. 96). Perform them at least three times this week, preferably on each other even if only one of you is experiencing pain.

Begin an initial ergonomic assessment of your workspace.

Week 2

Review your results from Week 1: Were the techniques helpful? Do you both feel as though you were doing them correctly?

Start your diary, looking for analogous movements you will use to reverse the effects of the learned neurological response.

Continue to evaluate your workspace.

Introduce the next two techniques (p. 98 and p. 100).

Week 3

Again, begin with a weekly review. If you have been doing the techniques consistently, by now you should be comfortable with performing the techniques you have started with, and will get a sense of their potential efficacy.

Take an hour and address some of the issues you have identified in your workspace.

Introduce Techniques 5 (p. 102) and 6 (p. 104).

Introduce some of the analogous movements you have identified in your diary along with the pain-inducing movements, as described in "The Learned Neurological Response: Teaching an Old Dog New Tricks" (p. 58).

Week 4

If you have not been exercising, introduce some form of movement three to five times a week (a brief walk will do). If you have been working out, this would be a great time to take it up a notch—add a new activity, increase your time on the treadmill or bike, or increase the resistance on the weight machines. It does not matter what you do, as long as you are taking steps to increase your strength and endurance.

Add Techniques 7 (p. 106) and 8 (p. 108).

At the end of the first month, celebrate! You two have actually taken steps towards feeling better. You and your partner should go out to dinner, relax, enjoy yourselves, and feel the gratitude that comes from helping each other. You have accomplished a lot at this point and you deserve a reward for your efforts.

Now you have some idea of what an implementation plan should look like. Obviously, you both need to do frequent reassessments, refer back to your journals, and continually update and fine-tune your own personal programs.

Sample Journal Entry

Week # and Date	Regions of Body	Techniques and # of times	Partner A's Comments	Partner B's Comments	Goals for next seesion

A Cautionary Tale: Mike and Sarah

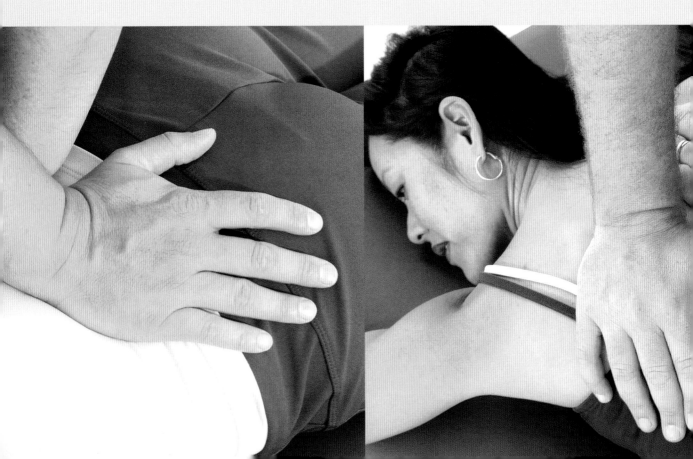

I have been doing private *Back Together* assessments for several years. For about three thousand dollars, I perform an ergonomic assessment of a couple's home and workspace, review a lot of the information I have provided in this book, and teach them, one on two, how to perform the pertinent hands-on techniques for their individual pain situations. Most of the time, these direct home interventions are very effective in jumpstarting the recovery process. The response has been overwhelmingly positive.

That is why I found this couple so interesting.

Mike and Sarah had gone back and forth about whether they should spend the money to have the *Back Together* private program in their own home. I did not want to push them too hard, as I was the one who stood to profit.

They deliberated intensely for about three months and decided to get the program. I went to their home and gave them what was in my opinion a great private workshop. For their money, they received an entire day of direct instruction, preceded by about four days of preliminary assessment and preparatory work. (I always want people to feel that they get their money's worth.)

Built into the cost of my program is an intensive post-course follow-up, usually at one month and three months. Because of their busy schedules, they had to forgo the one-month follow-up, and we got together for the three-month meeting.

When they sat down in my conference room, I expected them to tell me the same things that most couples I have worked with had—my program was helpful, they were **eternally indebted** to me, they planned to name their firstborn after me, and they would petition to have my face emblazoned on one of the state's quarters. So I was completely taken off guard when they told me that they had experienced no benefit whatsoever, and had even contemplated asking me for their money back.

I reviewed my notes from the previous meeting, and the specifics of the plan I laid out for them. I was really at a loss to explain why their results had been so utterly disappointing. Once I was confident that I had not left any serious holes in the plan we had developed, I began to talk to them about it in depth, in order to be certain that they understood the facets of the approach we had mutually agreed upon. When I was sure that they had really grasped the gist of my suggestions, I was truly at a loss. I was about to get my checkbook out and offer to return their fee. It was then that I had a revelation:

"Sarah," I asked, "how frequently are you doing the hands-on exercises with Mike?"

"We try to do them regularly," she replied.

"How regularly?"

"I would say we have done them at least three or four times."

"Mike," I continued, "how is that new desk chair working out?"

"I haven't assembled it yet—it only showed up a few weeks ago."

"And those workspace recommendations I made—your computer position, the monitor height and all that other stuff?"

"I was going to do that this weekend."

"Can I see the diary you've been keeping with your subjective pain ratings, and the things you've done?"

"I keep all of that in my head."

When you read this, you probably think I am making this up. I personally had thought that the large sum of money Mike and Sarah spent would be adequate motivation to actually *do* some of the things I had recommended.

When I began my investigation into the "self-help" genre, I spoke with people who had recommended some of the books I reviewed. After reading the books, I asked them which recommendations in them they had actually *acted upon*. It soon became obvious to me that while many of these books offered extremely good advice, hardly anybody actually did the things that the authors suggested. Additionally, the people who did follow up tended to do so only briefly, even when the recommendations were useful.

This realization was really upsetting.

I sent Mike and Sarah home (I kept their money), and gently encouraged them to do the activities, modifications, and procedures we had discussed in our meetings. All right, upon reflection I was probably not all that gentle about it; my encouragement probably sounded more like "Do the damn plan before I come to your home and MAKE you do it!"

They did. They felt better. So did I. (I was actually relieved; I had used the money from their consultation to buy the computer I used to write this book!)

Please attempt some of the suggestions and techniques I have described. They will most likely provide some benefit to you, and even if they do not, at least you will have tried. Many people derive a certain degree of satisfaction from buying books, tapes, and videos, and not even looking at them. A few people look at them and then ignore the advice they get. You will never, ever get better by osmosis. You will get better through your actions, and now you have some idea of the actions to take. Try to maintain a diary of them, and monitor your progress. When you reach a plateau, add something new to your approach.

What Does This All Mean?

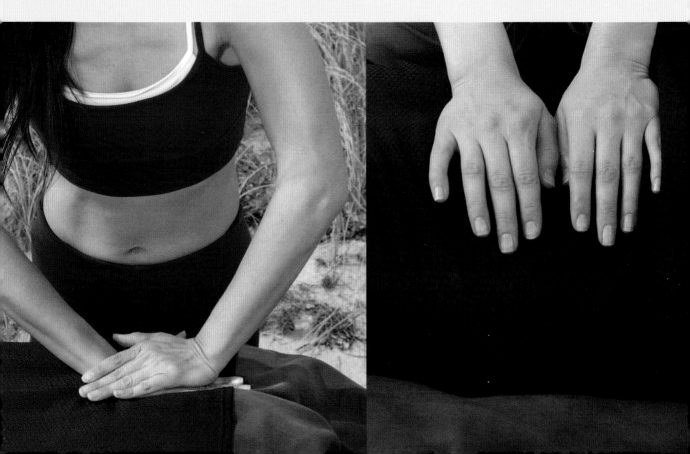

So many people are walking around in pain every day. You can tell by the way they walk, by the way they get out of a chair, by the expressions on their faces. There are many reasons people have back and neck pain: injuries, lifestyle factors, stress, just to name a few. Awareness of the basic causes of this pain and how they cross-pollinate with lifestyle factors is itself a tremendously powerful tool.

Now that you two have had an opportunity to examine some of the mechanisms that cause pain, it will be easier for both of you to understand and implement some of the strategies I have put forth for getting rid of the discomfort. The engineering feat nature has performed in the design and execution of the human spine is nothing short of astounding. Once we learn to appreciate the perfection of its design, and realize that things going wrong with it are often due to something that we have inflicted upon it, we can understand why these basic steps can go such a long way toward recovering a fantastic quality of life.

You need to know that you can control your outcome. You are an agent for your own well-being, and your actions and attitude will get you through to the other side. Having the assistance of a partner or loved one enriches the journey and can even make it fun!

As I related earlier, you may not experience a huge relief in your levels of pain by simply employing one or two of this book's techniques. When you make lifestyle changes, address some of the underlying mechanical issues causing your pain, and combine these with the techniques, you will begin to see a difference. Some of the lifestyle changes I suggest may seem drastic, but with time they should become second nature.

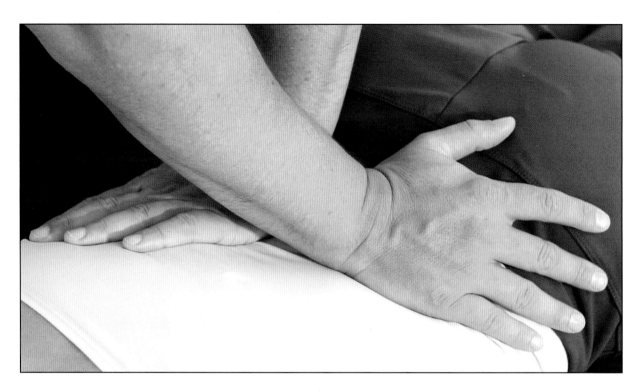

As I've said, many people will buy a book, take a course, or watch a video, but then take no action to follow up on what they have learned. That is another reason why a couples-based approach to pain is so effective. You can coach each other and make the effort together. The rewards will be enormous. I have seen the destructive power pain can have upon relationships, and you have probably felt some inkling of it as well. I have also seen the tremendous amounts of relief and mutual satisfaction that can be achieved when partners help each other to heal. Be there for each other.

Now that you've reached the end of this book, you should have confidence in the knowledge that pain cannot control you. *You* can take control. With practice, the hands-on techniques will become easy. When you use the information in this book to assert your newfound power, you will develop confidence in your capabilities.

Congratulations on completing some of your first steps toward feeling better. Again, I sincerely thank you for taking the time to listen to what I have to say. Be well.

You know, I guess this is a self-help book after all.

Dr. Andrew Kirschner, D.O., a board certified physician in family medicine and Osteopathic manual medicine, is the founder and medical director of Back Together, a program he has devised to teach safe, noninvasive, pain-relieving techniques to patients and their loved ones.

Back Together grew out of a need that arose during his wife's pregnancy. He and his wife, Donna, wondered whether some gentle manual medicine techniques would help alleviate the discomfort of pregnancy and the pain of childbirth. Dr. Kirschner experimented and developed his own. They were so effective, Donna remained comfortable during her pregnancy and had a relatively pain-free delivery. The ease of her labor and delivery inspired her to become a certified childbirth instructor.

Donna was so confident in the power of partner-based coaching to relieve pain that she urged her husband to teach his pain-relieving techniques to his own patients and their loved ones.

Andrew also maintains Kirschner Osteopathic, a private medical practice in Bala Cynwyd, Pa., which he designed to offer the most personalized care of its kind. The proprietary techniques he developed for Back Together grew out of his work dealing with the musculoskeletal pains of a broad cross-section of individuals—including athletes, performers, office workers, senior citizens, children and the physically challenged.

He has written and spoken extensively on the subjects of pain management, sports injuries and the seldom-addressed relationship issues of physical pain.

Andrew earned his Doctorate in Osteopathy from the Philadelphia College of Osteopathic Medicine, where he studied with some of the masters of Osteopathic manual medicine. A long-time Philadelphia resident, he lives in Bala Cynwyd, PA with his wife, Donna, and their daughter, Ella.